Pain in Rheumatic Diseases

Editor

MARIPAT CORR

RHEUMATIC DISEASE CLINICS OF NORTH AMERICA

www.rheumatic.theclinics.com

Consulting Editor
MICHAEL H. WEISMAN

May 2021 • Volume 47 • Number 2

ELSEVIER

1600 John F. Kennedy Boulevard ● Suite 1800 ● Philadelphia, Pennsylvania, 19103-2899
http://www.theclinics.com

RHEUMATIC DISEASE CLINICS OF NORTH AMERICA Volume 47, Number 2
May 2021 ISSN 0889-857X, ISBN 13: 978-0-323-83540-4

Editor: Lauren Boyle
Developmental Editor: Karen Solomon

Rheumatic Disease Clinics of North America (ISSN 0889-857X) is published quarterly by Elsevier Inc., 360 Park Avenue South, New York, NY 10010-1710. Months of issue are February, May, August, and November. Business and editorial offices: 1600 John F. Kennedy Boulevard, Suite 1800, Philadelphia, PA 19103-2899. Periodicals postage paid at New York, NY and additional mailing offices. Subscription prices are USD 362.00 per year for US individuals, USD 1000.00 per year for US institutions, USD 100.00 per year for US students and residents, USD 427.00 per year for Canadian individuals, USD 1045.00 per year for Canadian institutions, USD 100.00 per year for Canadian students/residents, USD 465.00 per year for international individuals, USD 1045.00 per year for international institutions, and USD 230.00 per year for foreign students/residents. To receive student/ resident rate, orders must be accompanied by name of affiliated institution, date of term, and the *signature* of program/residency coordinator on institution letterhead. Orders will be billed at individual rate until proof of status received. Foreign air speed delivery is included in all *Clinics* subscription prices. All prices are subject to change without notice. **POSTMASTER:** Send address changes to *Rheumatic Disease Clinics of North America,* Elsevier Health Sciences Division, Subscription Customer Service, 3251 Riverport Lane, Maryland Heights, MO 63043. **Customer Service: 1-800-654-2452 (US and Canada). From outside of the US and Canada: 314-447-8871. Fax: 314-447-8029. For print support, e-mail: JournalsCustomerService-usa@elsevier.com. For on-line support, e-mail: JournalsOnlineSupport-usa@elsevier.com.**

Reprints. For copies of 100 or more of articles in this publication, please contact the Commercial Reprints Department, Elsevier Inc., 360 Park Avenue South, New York, New York, 10010-1710; Tel.: +1-212-633-3874, Fax: +1-212-633-3820, and E-mail: reprints@elsevier.com.

Rheumatic Disease Clinics of North America is covered in *MEDLINE/PubMed (Index Medicus), Current Contents/Clinical Medicine, Science Citation Index, ISI/BIOMED,* and *EMBASE/Excerpta Medica.*

Printed in the United States of America.

Contributors

CONSULTING EDITOR

MICHAEL H. WEISMAN, MD
Professor of Medicine, Emeritus, Division of Rheumatology, Cedars-Sinai Medical Center, Distinguished Professor of Medicine, Emeritus, David Geffen School of Medicine, University of California, Los Angeles, California, USA

EDITOR

MARIPAT CORR, MD
Professor of Medicine, Division of Rheumatology, Allergy and Immunology, University of California, San Diego, La Jolla, California, USA

AUTHORS

FEDERICO BALAGUÉ, MD
Rheumatology Department, HFR Fribourg-hôpital Cantonal, Fribourg, Switzerland

MATTHEW T. BELL, BS
School of Medicine, St. Louis University, St Louis, Missouri, USA

DAVID G. BORENSTEIN, MD
Clinical Professor, Department of Medicine, The George Washington University Medical Center, Partner, Arthritis and Rheumatism Associates, Washington, DC, USA

RATNESH CHOPRA, MD
Assistant Professor, Division of Rheumatology, UMass Medical School, Worcester, Massachusetts, USA

DANIEL JOSEPH CLAUW, MD
Professor of Anesthesiology, Medicine (Rheumatology) and Psychiatry, Director of Chronic Pain and Fatigue Research Center, The University of Michigan, Ann Arbor, Michigan, USA

MEGAN E.B. CLOWSE, MD
Division of Rheumatology and Immunology, Duke University Medical Center, Durham, North Carolina, USA

MARIPAT CORR, MD
Professor of Medicine, Division of Rheumatology, Allergy and Immunology, University of California, San Diego, La Jolla, California, USA

LAURIANE DELAY, PhD
Department of Anesthesiology, University of California, San Diego, La Jolla, California, USA

ELAYNE VIEIRA DIAS, PhD
Department of Anesthesiology, University of California, San Diego, La Jolla, California, USA

BRETT W. DIETZ, MD
Division of Rheumatology, Department of Medicine, University of California, San Francisco, San Francisco, California, USA

AMANDA M. EUDY, PhD
Division of Rheumatology and Immunology, Duke University Medical Center, Durham, North Carolina, USA

GILSON GONÇALVES DOS SANTOS, PhD
Department of Anesthesiology, University of California, San Diego, La Jolla, California, USA

OLIVER HULLAND, MD
Department of Emergency Medicine, Yale-New Haven Hospital, Yale University, New Haven, Connecticut, USA

ROBERT D. INMAN, MD, FRCPC, FACP, FRCP Edin
Spondylitis Program, Schroeder Arthritis Institute, University Health Network, Departments of Medicine and Immunology, University of Toronto, Toronto, Ontario, Canada

PRIYANKA IYER, MBBS, MPH
Clinical Assistant Professor, Division of Rheumatology, Department of Internal Medicine, University of California, Irvine, Irvine, California, USA

NANCY E. LANE, MD
Professor of Medicine, Rheumatology, and Aging Research, Division of Rheumatology, Department of Internal Medicine, UC Davis Health, Sacramento, California, USA

YVONNE C. LEE, MD, MMSc
Associate Professor of Medicine and Preventative Medicine, Northwestern University, Chicago, Illinois, USA

ANNE-MARIE MALFAIT, MD, PhD
Department of Internal Medicine, Division of Rheumatology, Rush University Medical Center, Chicago, Illinois, USA

ALEXANDER MARTIN, MD
Fellow, Division of Rheumatology, UMass Medical School, Worcester, Massachusetts, USA

RACHEL E. MILLER, PhD
Department of Internal Medicine, Division of Rheumatology, Rush University Medical Center, Chicago, Illinois, USA

RICHARD J. MILLER, PhD
Department of Pharmacology, Northwestern University, Chicago, Illinois, USA

DEEBA MINHAS, MD
Clinical Lecturer, Department of Internal Medicine, Division of Rheumatology, University of Michigan, Ann Arbor, Michigan, USA

MARY C. NAKAMURA, MD
Professor of Medicine, Division of Rheumatology, Department of Medicine, University of California, San Francisco, San Francisco Veteran's Affairs Health Care System, San Francisco, California, USA

PERRY M. NICASSIO, PhD
Clinical Professor, Department of Psychiatry, University of California, Los Angeles, Los Angeles, California, USA

JESSICA OSWALD, MD, MPH
Associate Physician Pain Medicine, Center for Pain Medicine, Department of Anesthesiology, Associate Physician Emergency Medicine, Department of Emergency Medicine, UC San Diego Health, La Jolla, California, USA

EJAZ M.I. PATHAN, MD, PhD, MRCP
Consultant Rheumatologist, Rheumatology Department, Freeman Hospital, Newcastle upon Tyne Hospitals NHS Foundation Trust, Newcastle upon Tyne, United Kingdom

DAVID S. PISETSKY, MD, PhD
Professor of Medicine and Immunology, Division of Rheumatology and Immunology, Duke University Medical Center, Medical Research Service, Durham Veterans Administration Medical Center, Durham, North Carolina, USA

JENNIFER L. ROGERS, MD
Division of Rheumatology and Immunology, Duke University Medical Center, Durham, North Carolina, USA

TONY L. YAKSH, PhD
Department of Anesthesiology, University of California, San Diego, La Jolla, California, USA

Contents

Foreword: Pain in Rheumatic Diseases   xi

Michael H. Weisman

Preface: Pain in Rheumatic Diseases   xiii

Maripat Corr

Pain Mechanisms in Patients with Rheumatic Diseases   133

Deeba Minhas and Daniel Joseph Clauw

Patients with rheumatic diseases often have mixed pain states, with varying degrees of nociceptive, neuropathic, and nociplastic mechanisms, which exist on a continuum. When individuals with any chronic pain have a nociplastic component to their symptoms, they are less likely to respond to treatments (eg, injections, surgery, biologics, and opioids) that work better for acute or purely nociceptive pain.

Low Back Pain in Adolescent and Geriatric Populations   149

David G. Borenstein and Federico Balagué

Spinal pain is the most common form of musculoskeletal pain. Chronic low back pain may contain nociceptive, neuropathic, and central components. Children are at risk of developing spinal pain. An increasing proportion of children develop low back pain as they become adolescents. In most adolescents, no specific diagnosis is identified. Psychological factors play a role in adolescents with back pain. Lumbar spinal stenosis causes neurogenic claudication in older patients. Magnetic resonance imaging is the best radiographic technique to detect nerve compression. Surgical decompression with or without fusion may offer greater short-term benefit but may not be significantly better than medical therapy.

Basic Mechanisms of Pain in Osteoarthritis: Experimental Observations and New Perspectives   165

Anne-Marie Malfait, Rachel E. Miller, and Richard J. Miller

The specific changes in the peripheral neuronal pathways underlying joint pain in osteoarthritis are the focus of this review. The plasticity of the nociceptive system in osteoarthritis and how this involves changes in the structural, physiologic, and genetic properties of neurons in pain pathways are discussed. The role of the neurotrophin, nerve growth factor, in these pathogenic processes is discussed. Finally, how neuronal pathways are modified by interaction with the degenerating joint tissues they innervate and with the innate immune system is considered. These extensive cellular interactions provide a substrate for identification of targets for osteoarthritis pain.

Targeting Nerve Growth Factor for Pain Management in Osteoarthritis—Clinical Efficacy and Safety   181

Brett W. Dietz, Mary C. Nakamura, Matthew T. Bell, and Nancy E. Lane

Nerve growth factor (NGF) is a neurotrophin that mediates pain sensitization in pathologic states, including osteoarthritis. In clinical trials, antibodies to NGF reduce pain and improve physical function due to osteoarthritis of the knee or hip and have a long duration of action. Rapidly progressive osteoarthritis is a dose-dependent adverse event with these agents, and additional joint safety signals, such as subchondral insufficiency fractures and increased rates of total joint replacement, are reported. The effects on pain and potential mechanisms behind these joint events both are of considerable importance in the consideration of future use of anti-NGF therapies for osteoarthritis.

Pain in Axial Spondyloarthritis: Insights from Immunology and Brain Imaging   197

Ejaz M.I. Pathan and Robert D. Inman

Inflammatory back pain is characteristic of spondyloarthritis (SpA); however, this pain may not respond to treatment with NSAIDs or biologics. Pain is multifactorial and a combination of mechanical and inflammatory factors. A growing body of literature examines the impact of emotions on pain in SpA; many patients with this condition suffer from depression and fibromyalgia. Advanced imaging techniques can investigate the interplay of various brain networks in pain perception. Animal models have helped understand the interplay between the immune and nervous systems in pain generation and have highlighted differences in pain perception between the sexes.

The Categorization of Pain in Systemic Lupus Erythematosus   215

David S. Pisetsky, Amanda M. Eudy, Megan E.B. Clowse, and Jennifer L. Rogers

Systemic lupus erythematous is a systemic autoimmune disease that can cause severe pain and impair quality of life. Pain in lupus can arise from a variety of mechanisms and is usually assessed in terms of activity and damage. In contrast, categorization of symptoms as type 1 and type 2 manifestations encompasses a broader array of symptoms, including widespread pain, fatigue, and depression that may track together. The categorization of symptoms as type 1 and type 2 manifestations can facilitate communication between patient and provider as well as provide a framework to address more fully the complex symptoms experienced by patients.

Why It Hurts: The Mechanisms of Pain in Rheumatoid Arthritis   229

Priyanka Iyer and Yvonne C. Lee

Pain is a near-universal feature of rheumatoid arthritis, but peripheral joint inflammation may not suffice to explain the etiology of pain in all patients with rheumatoid arthritis. Inflammation in rheumatoid arthritis releases several algogens that may generate pain. Also, central nervous system processes may play a crucial role in the regulation and perpetuation of pain. Several methods for assessing pain in rheumatoid arthritis exist, and recently the role of assessing therapeutics in treating specific etiologies of pain has gained interest.

Sexual Dimorphism in the Expression of Pain Phenotype in Preclinical Models of Rheumatoid Arthritis   245

Lauriane Delay, Gilson Gonçalves dos Santos, Elayne Vieira Dias, Tony L. Yaksh, and Maripat Corr

Rheumatoid arthritis is one of most frequent rheumatic diseases, affecting around 1% of the population worldwide. Pain impacting the quality of life for the patient with rheumatoid arthritis, is often the primary factor leading them to seek medical care. Although sex-related differences in humans and animal models of rheumatoid arthritis are described, the correlation between pain and sex in rheumatoid arthritis has only recently been directly examined. Here we review the literature and explore the mechanisms underlying the expression of the pain phenotype in females and males in preclinical models of rheumatoid arthritis.

Cannabinoids and Pain: The Highs and Lows   265

Oliver Hulland and Jessica Oswald

The medicolegal landscape of cannabis continues to change, and with ever increasing access there has been a concurrent proliferation of research seeking to understand the utility of cannabinoids in treating innumerable conditions with pain at the forefront. This article seeks to summarize clinically relevant findings in cannabinoid research to better prepare clinicians in the utility of cannabis in the treatment of pain.

Nonpharmacologic Pain Management in Inflammatory Arthritis   277

Alexander Martin, Ratnesh Chopra, and Perry M. Nicassio

This article provides an overview of nonpharmacologic options for the treatment of pain in patients with inflammatory arthritis, such as peripheral spondyloarthritis, psoriatic arthritis, ankylosing spondylitis, and rheumatoid arthritis. The experience of pain in chronic disease is a complex process influenced by multiple domains of health. The discussion focuses on the establishment of a framework for pain control that engages with factors that influence the experience of pain and explores the evidence base that supports specific modalities of nonpharmacologic pain control, such as mindfulness, cognitive behavioral therapy, exercise, massage, splinting, and heat therapy. Rheumatoid and spondyloarthritides are considered separately.

RHEUMATIC DISEASE CLINICS OF NORTH AMERICA

FORTHCOMING ISSUES

August 2021
Lupus
Alfred Kim and Zahi Touma, *Editors*

November 2021
Pediatric Rheumatology Part I
Laura E. Schanberg and Yukiko Kimura, *Editors*

February 2022
Pediatric Rheumatology Part II
Laura E. Schanberg and Yukiko Kimura, *Editors*

RECENT ISSUES

February 2021
Health Disparities in Rheumatic Diseases: Part II
Candace H. Feldman, *Editor*

November 2020
Health Disparities in Rheumatic Diseases: Part I
Candace H. Feldman, *Editor*

August 2020
Cancer and Rheumatic Diseases
John Manley Davis, *Editor*

SERIES OF RELATED INTEREST

Medical Clinics of North America
https://www.medical.theclinics.com/
Neurologic Clinics
https://www.neurologic.theclinics.com/
Dermatologic Clinics
https://www.derm.theclinics.com/
Physical Medicine and Rehabilitation Clinics of North America
https://www.pmr.theclinics.com/

THE CLINICS ARE AVAILABLE ONLINE!
Access your subscription at:
www.theclinics.com

Foreword

Pain in Rheumatic Diseases

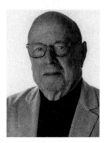

Michael H. Weisman, MD
Consulting Editor

Dr Maripat Corr has put together a remarkable "theme" issue about pain, a real tour de force! Since pain is what distinguishes our patients from almost all other disciplines and specialties and in most cases also drives our clinical and therapeutic decisions, we appreciate the opportunity to receive this information in order to understand the complex nature of pain in rheumatic diseases. The conditions we deal with are also challenging since even in a single patient there may be more than one pain mechanism or experience. Dr Corr tells us that the research efforts, contained herein, are an attempt to unravel the various pain mechanisms among which are tissue inflammation and damage, nerve damage, and central sensitization. The drugs that we use to target these areas are often accompanied by an incomplete understanding of the mechanism of action of many of them. Dr Corr chose to develop articles with specificity toward the more common rheumatic diseases, such as osteoarthritis, rheumatoid arthritis, ankylosing spondylitis, and systemic lupus erythematosus. Our often empiric approaches to pain in these diseases have driven us to employ management strategies that clearly are in advance of our understanding of the mechanisms involved, including the role of cell signaling, pain pathways, and innate immune networks. The conundrum of central pain sensitization is discussed with the appropriate clinical strategies regarding management as well as diagnosis. Finally, there is the issue of pain management for conditions that are defined by pain itself; we have been challenged by the use of opiates and cannabinoids that become part of the polypharmacy related to comorbid conditions that by themselves may be part of the problem. As our tools have grown to engage new research opportunities, so have the clinical insights provided by our

Rheum Dis Clin N Am 47 (2021) xi–xii
https://doi.org/10.1016/j.rdc.2021.02.002
0889-857X/21/© 2021 Published by Elsevier Inc.

authors and Dr Corr that are in evidence from this remarkable, timely, and very welcome issue.

Michael H. Weisman, MD
Division of Rheumatology
Cedars-Sinai Medical Center
8700 Beverly Boulevard
Los Angeles, CA 90048, USA

E-mail address:
michael.weisman@cshs.org

Preface

Pain in Rheumatic Diseases

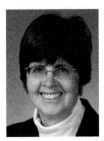

Maripat Corr, MD
Editor

The 5 classic signs of inflammation include redness (Latin rubor), pain (dolor), heat (calor), swelling (tumor), and loss of function. Hence, it is not surprising that pain would be a frequent concern of patients with rheumatic diseases. The mechanisms associated with pain perception are complex and involve both central and peripheral processes associated with nociception coupled with responses to individualized experiences, such as sleep disturbances, psychosocial stresses, and past circumstances. Although there have been exciting advances in the treatments of inflammation with an increasing number of targeted therapies, it has become clear that the clinical resolution of redness, warmth, and swelling may not be accompanied by complete relief of pain. Recent advances in imaging technology, clinical assessment tools, and animal models are providing new insights into this issue.

In this issue, important clinical and mechanistic questions are addressed across major areas that affect patients with rheumatic diseases. In the introductory article by Minhas and Clauw, current concepts of pain mechanisms are reviewed. The authors note that patients often have mixed pain states, and Minhas and Clauw provide a basic framework for clinicians to deconvolute components of nociceptive pain (due to tissue damage or inflammation), neuropathic pain (associated with nerve damage and dysfunction), and nociplastic pain (central sensitization). This last component of pain is least likely to respond to medications that treat inflammation or nociceptive pain and presents interesting challenges. These principles apply to adolescents as well geriatric patients. Borenstein and Balagué discuss recent data regarding spinal pain, the most common form of musculoskeletal pain, with an emphasis on younger and older populations. Symptoms of back pain are increasing among adolescents, and the older population is at risk for developing spinal stenosis. Diagnostic strategies and short- and long-term treatment outcomes are presented.

Given the complexities of pain, in vitro experimental approaches have been limited in developing our understanding of the intercellular signaling networks, and animal

Rheum Dis Clin N Am 47 (2021) xiii–xv
https://doi.org/10.1016/j.rdc.2021.02.001
0889-857X/21/© 2021 Published by Elsevier Inc.

models have provided additional insights. Dos Santos and colleagues outline studies that concurrently assess the painlike behaviors in male and female rodents in inflammatory arthritis models. There are clear mechanistic differences between the sexes that are only partially explained by sex hormones and their receptors. Malfait and colleagues review specific changes in the peripheral neuronal pathways underlying joint pain in osteoarthritis. They provide perspectives on the plasticity of the nociceptive system in osteoarthritis, and the associated changes in the structural, physiologic, and genetic properties of neurons in related pain pathways. The authors posit that the changes in neurons that interact with the innate immune system and innervate degenerative joints may lead to the identification of additional treatment targets for osteoarthritis and other pathologic conditions that manifest as arthralgias.

Beyond the categorization of global pain states, specific diseases can also contribute to our overall understanding. Three articles summarize the current knowledge base in relation to pain for systemic lupus erythematosus, rheumatoid arthritis, and ankylosing spondylitis. Pisetsky and colleagues discuss the mechanisms of pain arising in lupus and describe the advantages of categorizing symptoms as 2 types of manifestations of pain in the context of other symptoms, including fatigue and depression. This approach may be useful in addressing complex symptoms in a patient-centered manner. Iyer and Lee outline the mechanisms that lead to central pain sensitization in rheumatoid arthritis and the perpetuation of pain with minimal or no nociceptive stimulation. Quantitative sensory testing and neuroimaging methods to study different components of pain in rheumatoid arthritis and their use in assessing therapeutics are also discussed. The interaction of immune cells and neurons also plays a role in the development and perpetuation of pain perception in ankylosing spondylitis. Pathon and Inman present how advanced imaging techniques have been used to investigate the interplay of various brain networks in the perception of pain. These networks exhibit functional connectivity, which modulates pain perception in ankylosing spondylitis. Imaging and other studies that demonstrate sexual dimorphism in pain perceptions are also discussed.

In the United States, there has been mounting concern surrounding the long-term use of opioids for chronic pain. Clearly new treatment strategies are needed, particularly for nociplastic pain. Three articles examine different facets of potential treatment strategies. Dietz and colleagues focus on the benefits and risks of targeted therapies that block nerve growth factor, a neurotropin that mediates pain in a variety of pathologic conditions, including cancer and osteoarthritis. The promising data from recent clinical trials demonstrating long-term pain relief are presented, and the caveats of safety signals for rapidly progressive osteoarthritis and enhanced risk with concurrent use of nonsteroidal anti-inflammatory drugs are discussed. Although cannabinoids are not necessarily a new therapeutic class, Hulland and Oswald present the utility of cannabinoids in treating painful conditions following recent changes in the medicolegal landscape. This article outlines the need for high-quality data to guide clinicians in the use of this therapy. It would be remiss to assume that all therapeutic strategies exclusively involve injections and tablets. Martin and colleagues provide an overview of nonpharmacologic options for the treatment of pain in patients with inflammatory arthritis, such as psoriatic arthritis, ankylosing spondylitis, and rheumatoid arthritis. These authors explore the evidence that supports specific modalities of nonpharmacologic pain control, such as mindfulness, cognitive behavioral therapy, exercise, massage, splinting, and heat therapy. They seek to provide the practitioner with a framework for pain control that addresses factors that influence the experience of pain.

Clinical and basic science research has advanced our understanding of the complexities of different pain states. Clearly, as diagnostic, imaging, and molecular tools continue to improve, new opportunities for clinical insights and applications are emerging. Here, I invite the readers on behalf of the authors to use these articles to incorporate a new understanding of the complexities of pain experienced by patients and enhance our treatment approaches with a new eye toward what is likely the most compelling issue for our patients.

Maripat Corr, MD
University of California San Diego
9500 Gilman Drive
La Jolla, CA 92093-0663, USA

E-mail address:
mpcorr@health.ucsd.edu

Pain Mechanisms in Patients with Rheumatic Diseases

Deeba Minhas, MD[a], Daniel Joseph Clauw, MD[b],*

KEYWORDS

- Nociplastic • Central sensitization • Rheumatic pain • Pain mechanisms

KEY POINTS

- Pain in rheumatic disorders can occur via any combination of 3 mechanisms: nociceptive pain (tissue damage and inflammation), neuropathic pain (nerve damage and dysfunction), and a new category of pain—nociplastic pain.
- Nociplastic pain (best exemplified by fibromyalgia) often is superimposed on and is independent of the other 2 mechanisms.
- Nociplastic pain is driven by the central nervous system, especially involving augmented pain and sensory processing.
- In the rheumatic diseases, ongoing nociceptive input can cause central sensitization, or nociplastic pain. This component of pain is less likely to respond to medications that treat nociceptive pain.

INTRODUCTION

Pain in the rheumatic diseases traditionally has been characterized as solely nociceptive, implying that targeting inflammation should manage rheumatic pain effectively. Despite therapeutic advancements providing excellent control of inflammation, however, patients continue to have pain. It is now known that pain is complex, with varying components of nociceptive, neuropathic, and a new type—nociplastic—pain, which is driven by augmented central nervous system (CNS) processing. These can occur in isolation, or represent a mixed pain picture, with substantial overlap in mechanisms.

Nociceptive Pain

Nociceptive pain results from tissue damage caused by trauma, nonhealing injury, or inflammatory processes. It is the primary type of pain in patients with rheumatic diseases and musculoskeletal disorders with underlying structural pathology.[1]

[a] Department of Internal Medicine, Division of Rheumatology, University of Michigan, Ann Arbor, MI, USA; [b] The University of Michigan, 24 Frank Lloyd Wright Drive Lobby M, Ann Arbor, MI 48106, USA
* Corresponding author.
E-mail address: dclauw@med.umich.edu

Rheum Dis Clin N Am 47 (2021) 133–148
https://doi.org/10.1016/j.rdc.2021.01.001
0889-857X/21/© 2021 Elsevier Inc. All rights reserved.
rheumatic.theclinics.com

Neuropathic Pain

Neuropathic pain typically is manifested as electric shock-like, lancinating, aching, numbing, burning, or tingling sensations that are distinct from nociceptive pain. It is the direct result of lesions or diseases of the somatosensory nervous system.[2]

Peripheral and Central Sensitization

When activated by noxious stimuli, local nociceptors secrete hundreds of inflammatory and proalgesic signaling molecules and convert to nerve signals in first-order somatosensory Aδ-nociceptor and C-nociceptor afferent terminals in the periphery. These nerve signals then are transmitted via specialized nerve fibers to the dorsal horn of the spinal cord and ascending cortical pathways to the brain.[3,4] Chemical mediators and neuropeptides are released and reduce the threshold for nociceptor neurons to generate action potentials, leading to amplified responsiveness and ultimately heightened pain sensitivity—termed, *peripheral sensitization*.[5]

This is a local, self-limited, protective mechanism and resolves as tissues heal and inflammation recedes.[6] If the stimuli are prolonged, neuroplastic changes of the nociceptors in the CNS at spinal and/or supraspinal levels occur; this is termed, *central sensitization*.[7,8]

Nociplastic Pain

The International Association for the Study of Pain now has referred to centralized pain as nociplastic pain.[9] Symptoms originate from augmented CNS pain and sensory processing and it is mechanistically different from nociceptive or neuropathic pain (**Table 1**). Hallmarks are diffuse hyperalgesia (increased pain to normally painful stimuli) and allodynia (pain to normally nonpainful stimuli). Along with chronic widespread pain (CWP), CNS-derived symptoms, for example, fatigue, mood disturbances, cognitive dysfunction, memory issues, and nonrestorative sleep, can occur. Perceptual amplification of auditory stimuli, along with increased sensitivity to complex visual stress light and unpleasant odors, also are noted; the auditory and visual sensitivities often are correlated with pain sensitivity in these patients.[10]

Nociplastic Pain Syndromes

A wide spectrum of pain disorders has been identified, with varying degrees of the contribution of nociplastic mechanisms.[11] The National Institutes of Health recently coined the term, *chronic overlapping pain conditions* (COPCs), to characterize the nociplastic pain syndromes, including fibromyalgia (FM), chronic fatigue syndrome, irritable bowel syndrome, interstitial cystitis, vulvodynia, endometriosis, chronic migraine and tension-type headache, nonspecific chronic low back pain, and temporomandibular disorders.[12] Pain may be activated by no identifiable inputs or normally benign inputs, with no particular abnormalities found on clinical examination, laboratory tests, and imaging.

Endophenotypes of Central Sensitization

COPCs are the prototypical example of a top-down, centralized pain state. The augmented pain and sensory processing in the CNS are characterized by a lifelong history of multifocal pain, multiple chronic pain conditions, high rates of comorbid symptoms, and familial predominance. Psychological contributors, such as depression and anxiety, are top-down sensitizers. Because emerging evidence suggests that therapies that work best for peripheral, nociceptive pain (eg, nonsteroidal anti-inflammatory drugs [NSAIDs], opioids, injections, and surgical procedures) are less

Table 1
Mechanistic characterization of pain

	Nociceptive	Neuropathic	Nociplastic
Cause	Inflammation or damage	Nerve damage or entrapment	CNS or systemic problem
Clinical features	Pain is well localized, consistent effect of activity on pain	Follows distribution of peripheral nerves (ie, dermatome or stocking/glove), episodic, lancinating, numbness, tingling	Pain is widespread and accompanied by fatigue, sleep, memory, and/or mood difficulties as well as history of previous pain elsewhere in body
Screening tools		painDETECT	Body map or FM survey
Treatment	NSAIDs, injections, surgery, ? opioids	Local treatments aimed at nerve (surgery, injections, topical) or CNS-acting drugs	CNS-acting drugs, nonpharmacological therapies
Classic examples	OA Autoimmune disorders Cancer pain	Diabetic painful neuropathy Postherpetic neuralgia Sciatica, carpal tunnel syndrome	FM Functional gastrointestinal disorders Temporomandibular disorder Tension headache Interstitial cystitis, bladder pain syndrome

Variable degrees of any mechanism can contribute in any disease.

Chronic pain can originate from 3 different sources: peripheral nociceptive input, such as damage or inflammation of tissues; nerve damage and dysfunction in neuropathic pain; and nociplastic pain with central spinal and supraspinal mechanisms. The central factors can be best thought of as volume control or pain setting on what happens to peripheral nociceptive input.

likely to be effective in these individuals,[13] it is important to address these contributors.

Bottom-up, central sensitization is driven by persistent nociceptive input.[14] **Fig. 1** highlights the distinctions. Recent studies have demonstrated that 18% to 24% of patients with inflammatory arthritis meet criteria for FM.[15] These estimates likely underestimate the co-occurrence of nociplastic pain in the form of subthreshold FM that commonly is seen and is associated with the characteristic clinical, quantitative sensory testing (QST), and neurobiological features of FM.[16,17] This does not mean that ongoing peripheral nociceptive input is not contributing to an individual's pain; instead, pain mechanisms are considered additive. Even COPCs can be mixed pain states, with components of all 3 mechanisms.

RISK FACTORS

The complex interaction of biologic, psychological, and behavioral mechanisms plays a prominent role in pain and symptom expression in all rheumatic diseases and complicates their treatment. For example, in rheumatoid arthritis (RA) and osteoarthritis (OA), education level, coping strategies, and socioeconomic variables account for more of the variance in pain and disability than joint narrowing or erythrocyte sedimentation rate.[18]

Mood

There is a strong bidirectional link between mood disorders and persistent pain. Rheumatic diseases have a high rate of comorbid depressive symptoms, ranging from 8% to 75% in a recent review.[19] Depression, anxiety, and negative affect, are the most

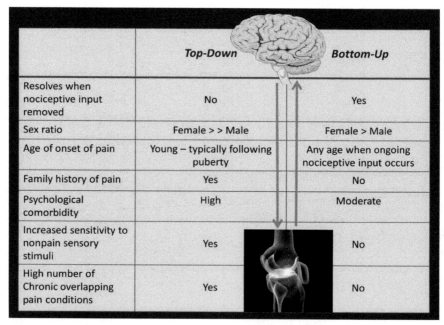

	Top-Down	Bottom-Up
Resolves when nociceptive input removed	No	Yes
Sex ratio	Female > > Male	Female > Male
Age of onset of pain	Young – typically following puberty	Any age when ongoing nociceptive input occurs
Family history of pain	Yes	No
Psychological comorbidity	High	Moderate
Increased sensitivity to nonpain sensory stimuli	Yes	No
High number of Chronic overlapping pain conditions	Yes	No

Fig. 1. Differences between top-down and bottom-up forms of central sensitization. (*Adapted from* Harte, SE, Harris, RE, Clauw, DJ. The neurobiology of central sensitization. J Appl Behav Res. 2018; 23:e12137.)

potent and robust predictors of the transition from acute to chronic pain.[20] and are strongly associated with persistent pain, physical disability, and mortality, more so than even pain intensity.[21]

Environmental Stressors and Trauma

COPCs are found in higher rates in individuals who have had certain infections (eg, Epstein-Barr virus, Lyme disease, Q fever, and viral hepatitis), and physical trauma (eg, motor vehicle collision). It often is challenging to attribute any single exposure (eg, in medicolegal) to the development of COPCs, because there often are preexisting or co-occurring stressors. A majority of patients return to their baseline health. Tenuous housing, employment status, low educational levels, and low family income have been associated with chronic pain; financial or housing insecurity–related stress may promote aberrant pain processing.[22]

Adult veterans, combat exposure, and posttraumatic stress disorder have strong statistical associations with chronic pain and transition from acute to chronic pain.[23,24] Psychological, sexual, or physical abuse is associated with a 2-fold to 3-fold increase in the development of CWP; in a recent meta-analyses,[23] childhood abuse conferred a 97% increase in risk for having FM or COPCs in adulthood.[23]

Cognitive Factors

Catastrophizing is a cognitive and emotional response to pain consisting of magnification, rumination, and helplessness about the ability to manage pain (eg, "This is the worst pain," "I can think of nothing else," and "There's nothing I can do"). It is the single most significant pretreatment risk associated with poor treatment outcomes for pain-relieving interventions. It is associated with enhanced anterior insular cortex activation on functional magnetic resonance imaging (fMRI) and frequently co-occurs with maladaptive behaviors, for example, fear of movement.

Social Support

In patients with chronic pain conditions, broad social support has been associated with improved functioning. In contrast, high levels of solicitous responses of parents or partners have been linked with higher pain intensity and pain-related disability.

Racism

As race has been moved away from being considered genetics-based to a social construct that captures the impacts of racism,[25] several studies increasingly have found that racial discrimination is significantly related to pain intensity and severity in African American groups.[26]

Sleep

Inadequate or interrupted sleep results in impaired inhibitory mechanisms; poor sleep is a strong predictor of subsequent pain and is noted in 90% of FM patients. Pain and abnormal sleep are cyclical and cumulative, and the severity of sleep disturbance correlates with pain severity, reduced pain inhibition, and fatigue.[27] In studies, nonrestorative sleep was the strongest predictor of CWP.

Lifestyle Factors

Physical inactivity is a risk factor for the development of chronic pain and may alter the CNS exaggerate responses to low-intensity muscle insults. Smoking and consumption of high-fat foods have been linked to hyperalgesia.

Resilience and Protective Factors

Historically, the factors have been studied that make it more likely to develop pain but little attention has been paid to factors that might be protective. In many studies across many diseases, the presence of these protective factors often more powerfully predicts who will not develop chronic pain than negative factors predict who will. For example, positive affect and optimism are associated with lower pain sensitivity, lower pain intensity, and less dysfunction[28] Positive affect is thought to be a mediator of resilience, lowering pain catastrophizing, and may buffer maladaptive pain-related behaviors, such as fear of movement. Positive affect is surprisingly highly malleable; encouraging behavioral activation (having patients schedule and perform things they find enjoyable), aimed at raising positive feelings, cognitions, and behaviors rather than reducing negative ones, has shown large effect sizes with mood and improvements with chronic pain.

Encouraging lifestyle modification, cognitive-behavior therapy, and mind-body techniques, such as mindfulness, have been shown to have beneficial effects on chronic pain and pain-related outcomes. These techniques can improve patients' self-efficacy—individuals' belief in their ability to perform a behavior or achieve the desired outcome. This determines thoughts, feelings, and behaviors in stressful situations and affects the ability to successfully cope when confronted with challenges, specifically to increase pain self-efficacy.

Pain-related expectations also influence the experience of pain as well as treatment outcome, and learning active coping techniques (ie, techniques used to control pain or continue functioning despite the pain) is associated with positive outcomes, including positive affect, better psychological adjustment, and decreased depression.[21]

MECHANISTIC STUDIES
Quantitative Sensory Testing

QST is a method that identifies abnormalities in pain mechanisms by assessing pain in response to quantifiable noxious stimuli[29] and has been used in most early studies of nociplastic pain conditions. Data from QST studies suggest a wide, bell-shaped distribution in pain sensitivity across the general population.[30,31] Individuals with nociplastic pain syndromes fall on the right side of the curve, noting diffuse hypersensitivity in both at and outside the region of injury (ie, secondary hyperalgesia and allodynia).[30,32] This type of testing can be mechanistically elucidating in rheumatology, where disease measures for example, the Clinical Disease Activity Index (CDAI), which includes subjective components, for example, tender joint count (TJC) and patient global assessments (PGAs), may reflect higher disease inaccurately activity by underestimating the role of nociplastic pain.

Individuals with nociplastic pain are noted to have descending inhibitory pain pathways that do not function appropriately, as measured by conditioned modulation paradigms (CPMs). Impaired CPM also has been shown in RA patients with nociplastic pain, which may be mediated by sleep disturbances.[33]

Temporal summation (TS) is the clinical measure of windup—the progressive summation of C-fiber responses in response to repetitive noxious stimuli, leading to increased firing of the dorsal horn, leading to increasing perceived pain intensity.[34] This normal response, which occurs in healthy individuals, is enhanced in central sensitization and is predictive of individuals who will respond poorly to peripheral pain interventions.

The pain threshold is defined as the point at which a particular sensation first becomes painful. In studies of stable RA patients on disease-modifying antirheumatic drugs treatment, low pressure pain thresholds (PPTs) (high pain sensitivity) were associated with higher TJC, worse PGA, higher depression, and higher FM scores.[35] Lee and colleagues[17] demonstrated high pain sensitivity (low PPTs and high TS) was associated with high CDAI scores, supporting the role of nociplastic pain in RA.

QST studies have shown that FM patients are just as hyper-responsive to auditory, visual, and other sensory stimuli as they are to pain and that this is a key feature of this pain mechanism. The brain regions that are known to be hyperactive in nociplastic pain, for example, the insula, are involved in the processing of all sensory stimuli, not just painful stimuli.

Functional Brain Imaging Studies

Functional, structural, and chemical functional brain imaging studies have enriched the understanding of the rheumatic disease pain mechanisms. They allow assessment of activity at rest as when individuals are given stimuli (ie, evoked scans), and when used in combination in the same individual much can be gleamed regarding underlying neural mechanisms.

For instance, the insula consistently is hyperactive and likely to play a key pathogenic role. The insula displays differentiation; the posterior serves a purer sensory role, and the anterior is associated with the emotional processing of sensations.[36] The connectivity between the insula and the default mode network (DMN) (a group of interconnected brain regions, including the medial prefrontal cortex, posterior cingulate cortex, precuneus, inferior parietal lobule, hippocampal formation, and lateral temporal cortex) has attracted particular attention in recent years.[37] In healthy subjects, insula activity has no correlation with DMN regions. In chronic pain disorders, insula subregions can become functionally connected with the DMN; the degree of hyper-connectedness is related to ongoing pain severity.[38]

When individuals with FM are given a mild pressure or heat stimuli that most individuals feel as touch rather than pain, they experience pain and activation in pain-processing brain regions.[39,40] During a painful stimulus, connectivity is decreased between key anti-nociceptive regions (eg, the brainstem—the origin of descending analgesic pathways) and a brain region identified as a potential source of dysfunctional pain inhibition in FM.[41] Neuroimaging has confirmed QST studies that these individuals are more sensitive to several sensory stimuli other than pain, and machine learning paradigms can distinguish FM from non-FM patients accurately, with more than 90% accuracy using these results.[42,43]

Other neuroimaging techniques have been used to assess the levels of neurotransmitters and chemical mediators involved in driving nociplastic pain. Proton magnetic resonance spectroscopy can identify levels of excitatory neurotransmitters, for example, glutamate that typically are elevated in brain regions in FM,[43,44] Pregabalin and gabapentin work by reducing glutamatergic activity. Individuals with the highest pretreatment levels of glutamate in the posterior insula were those most likely to respond to pregabalin; the clinical response was associated with normalization of fMRI and connectivity findings.[44,45] Conversely, low levels of 1 of the body's major inhibitory neurotransmitters, γ-aminobutyric acid (GABA),[46,47] have been seen. This likely accounts for the effectiveness of GABAergic drugs, such as γ-hydroxybutyrate, in a subset of individuals with FM[48] and the observation that low amounts of alcohol might protect against the development of nociplastic pain.[49,50]

PET can examine binding of neurotransmitters in the CNS. A series of studies have found evidence of decreased mu-opioid receptor availability and increases in endogenous opioids in the cerebrospinal fluid of FM patients[51]—likely why opioids appear ineffective in FM. PET also recently has been used to identify possible evidence of glial cell activation in FM.[52]

Fig. 2 illustrates the neurotransmitters that have been demonstrated to influence pain transmission in the CNS. This neurochemical profile helps illustrate why no single class of CNS analgesia is likely to work in every patient with pain of CNS origin.

fMRI supports evidence that pain and depression largely are independent but overlapping physiologic processes in nociplastic pain. In FM, comorbid depression has been correlated with increased activity in the affective or motivational aspects of pain processing (mainly unpleasantness) regions—anterior insula and amygdala activations[53] but not associated with lateral brain structures involved in the sensory processing of pain (ie, location and intensity of the pain).

fMRI studies also have noted decreased activation in regions of the brain involved in sensory and emotional pain processing within 24 hours of tumor necrosis factor (TNF)-α inhibition in RA patients, potentially explaining the immediate pain relief noted.[54,55] Similar to other chronic pain syndromes, depressive symptoms in RA have been associated with activation of the medial prefrontal cortex[56] involved in emotional processing.

Genetics

The strong familial predisposition to nociplastic pain syndromes has prompted the search for specific genetic polymorphisms associated with pain processing. The

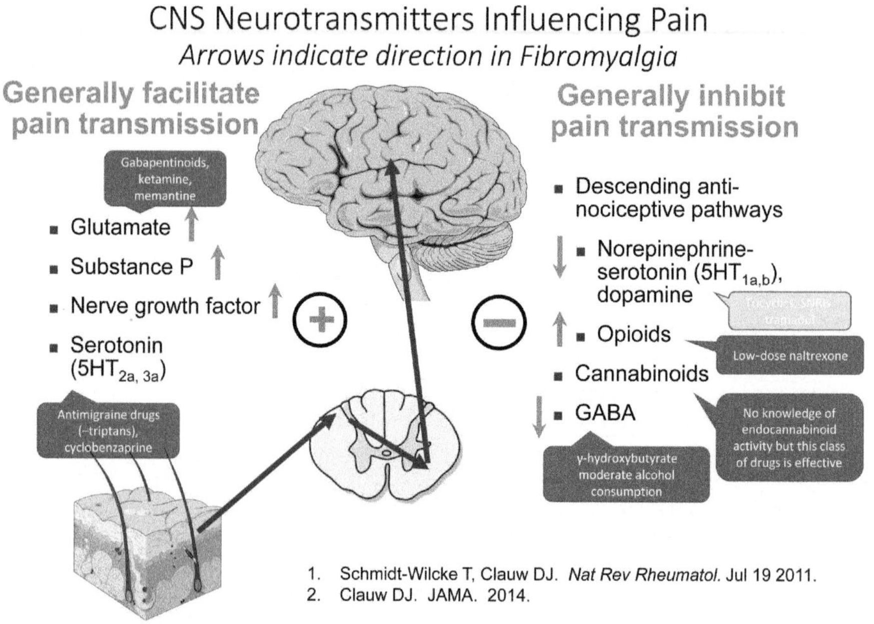

Fig. 2. Neurotransmitter systems that generally facilitate (*left*) or inhibit (*right*) CNS pain transmission. The arrows indicate the levels of these neurotransmitters in the CNS of individuals with FM, and the boxes indicate drugs that have been shown to be effective in FM that likely are working in part via those neurotransmitters. SNRI, serotonin-norepinephrine reuptake inhibitor. (Clauw, 2014; Schmidt-Wilcke and Clauw, 2011). (*Adapted from* Harte, SE, Harris, RE, Clauw, DJ. The neurobiology of central sensitization. J Appl Behav Res. 2018; 23:e12137.)

serotonin 5-HT2A receptor polymorphism T/T phenotype, serotonin transporter, dopamine-4-receptor, and catecholamine O-methyltransferase (COMT) polymorphisms all noted were in higher frequency in FM patients than controls, although this has not been replicated in subsequent studies.[57] The COMT gene encodes the enzyme believed to moderate the transmission of pain signals via the removal of catecholamine (ie, dopamine, epinephrine, and norepinephrine); reduced COMT activity appears to be related to increased pain sensitivity.[58] Currently, hundreds of genes thought to be relevant to human pain perception or analgesia have been identified, include the genes encoding voltage-gated sodium-channels (Nav), GTP cyclohydrolase 1, mu-opioid receptors, and various genes of the dopaminergic, glutamatergic, and GABAergic pathways.[59] Because environmental factors, for example, stress, influence pain pathogenesis, the role of epigenetics is being investigated.[60] Initial findings from chronic pain models suggest that chromatin structure alterations may trigger gene expression to promote the evolution from acute pain to central sensitization.[61]

The Role of Neuroendocrine or Autonomic Abnormalities

Because of this link between exposure to stressors and the subsequent development of nociplastic pain syndromes, the human stress systems have been studied extensively in this condition.[62] There have been inconsistencies in findings, and now it is posited that alterations of the hypothalamus-pituitary-adrenal (HPA) axis might represent a diathesis or be due to pain or early life stress, rather than causing it.

In 2 studies examining HPA function in FM, McLean and colleagues[63] showed that salivary cortisol levels varied with pain levels and that cerebrospinal fluid levels of

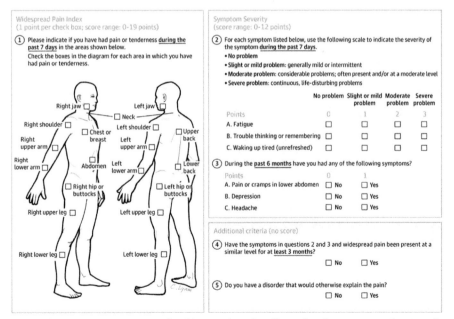

Fig. 3. The 2011 survey criteria for fibromyalgia (Wolfe and colleagues, 2011) using the Michigan Body Map (Brummett and colleagues, 2016). (*Adapted from* Harte, SE, Harris, RE, Clauw, DJ. The neurobiology of central sensitization. J Appl Behav Res. 2018; 23:e12137.)

corticotropin-releasing factor were related more closely to an individual's pain level or a history of early-life trauma than whether they were an FM case or control.

Evidence of Abnormal Cytokines and Immune Dysfunction in Nociplastic Pain

Although nociplastic pain is not thought to be autoimmune in nature, data suggest the immune system may be playing some role.[64] Multiple inhibitory transmitters act at the spinal level to reduce the volume of pain transmission, for example, serotonin, norepinephrine, enkephalins, dopamine, and GABA.

Animal models have found receptors for TNF-α, interleukin (IL-1β), and IL-17 on sensory neurons[65] and transmembrane signal-transducing subunit on the dorsal root ganglion neurons that binds to the IL-6/IL-6 receptor complex.[66] The most consistent finding noted to date is a mild elevation in IL-8, which is a cytokine associated with autonomic dysfunction; it could be related to the dysautonomia seen in some patients.[67] The roles of diet, obesity, and microglial involvement are being investigated actively.

The Role of Small Fiber Neuropathy in Nociplastic Pain

Although several groups have shown evidence of decreased intraepidermal nerve fiber density (ie, small fiber neuropathy) in FM,[68–71] the pathologic significance is unclear.[72] Reduced nerve fiber density is nonspecific, has been noted in more than 50

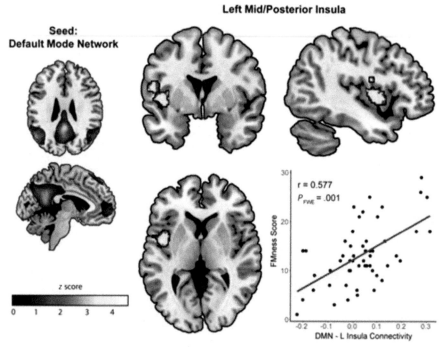

Fig. 4. Increased brain connectivity between the DMN and left mid/posterior insula in RA patients is associated with fibromyalgianess. Scatterplots show positive correlations for interindividual differences in brain connectivity (Fisher-transformed r values) with the total fibromyalgianess score. FEW, family-wise error. (*From* Basu N, Kaplan CM, Ichesco E, et al. Neurobiologic Features of Fibromyalgia Are Also Present Among Rheumatoid Arthritis Patients. Arthritis & Rheumatology. 2018;70(7):1000-1007.)

different pain and nonpain conditions,[72] and is reproducible in animal models of central sensitization, by increasing insular glutamate.[73] Reduced nerve fiber density likely reflects an adaptive structural and functional reorganization of the PNS in the context of ongoing chronic pain and neurologic conditions.

THE CONTINUUM OF FIBROMYALGIA TO FIBROMYALGIANESS

Wolfe[14] was the first to describe the concept and clinical importance of "fibromyalgianess" by showing that "subthreshold" FM amplifies the symptom severity in patients with rheumatologic and classically nociceptive diseases. In a series of studies, he showed that in individuals with conditions, such as RA, low back pain, and OA, an individual's FM score, derived with measures similar to the American College of Rheumatology 2010/2011/2016 FM criteria,[74] was more predictive of pain and disability than more objective measures of activity of these illnesses, such as measures of inflammation or joint damage.[75]

The entirely self-reported survey version assesses the Widespread Pain Index (up to 19 body areas each counted as 1 point) and the Symptom Severity Index (that queries

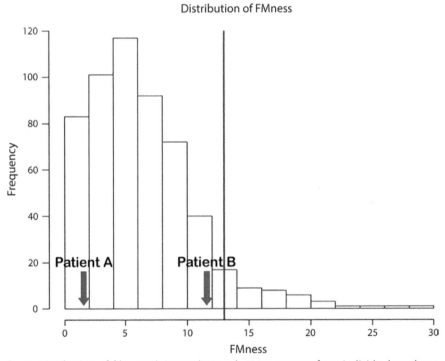

Fig. 5. Distribution of fibromyalgianess (FMness). FMness scores from individuals undergoing lower extremity arthroplasty for OA (Brummett and colleagues, 2013; Brummett and colleagues, 2015). The red line indicates the score meeting FM criteria. Two different hypothetical participants, without FM, are compared with respect to the amount of oral morphine equivalents required for pain control at 24 hours to 48 hours and the likelihood of achieving 50% improvement in pain at 6 months. Compared with Patient A with localized pain and no somatic symptoms, Patient B would need 90 mg more oral morphine equivalents during the first 48 hours of hospitalization, and is 5-times less likely to have a 50% improvement in pain at 6 months. (*Adapted from* Harte, SE, Harris, RE, Clauw, DJ. The neurobiology of central sensitization. J Appl Behav Res. 2018; 23:e12137.)

the presence and severity of fatigue, sleep disturbances, memory difficulties, each scored 0–3 for presence and severity) as well as irritable bowel, headaches, and mood problems (1 point each; total Symptom Severity Index score = 0–12). They are combined for a total FM score of 0 to 31, with a score of 13 as diagnostic of FM (**Fig. 3**).

The higher the score, the more nociplastic pain is contributing to patients' symptoms[14] and the more likely simply treating the nociceptive portion of the pain is not sufficient. This is supported further by a recent fMRI study by Basu and colleagues,[16] which found that increased connectivity between the DMN and the insula—the most consistently found feature of centralization in nociplastic pain syndromes— also was seen in RA patients with high degrees of fibromyalgianess (**Fig. 4**).

In a study by Brummett and colleagues, patients scheduled for hip or knee replacements or hysterectomies completed the 2011 FM survey criteria. For each 1-point increase in baseline FM score, individuals needed more morphine and had a 17.8% increase in the odds of failure to meet the threshold of 50% improvement in pain. This held true whether the score increased from 2 to 4 or from 12 to 14 (the latter score moving the individual into an FM diagnosis) (**Fig. 5**).

Recognizing superimposed nociplastic pain on top of nociceptive or neuropathic pain is essential, because the centralized component requires different treatment; peripherally directed treatments are not effective.

CLINICS CARE POINTS

- Many patients present with mixed pain states, with components of nociceptive pain, neuropathic pain, and nociplastic pain—or any combination of all 3.

- In addition to biologic and mechanical factors, psychological and behavioral mechanisms play a prominent role in pain and symptom expression in all rheumatic diseases and can have an impact on their treatment.

- Identifying potentially modifiable risk factors, such as physical inactivity and sleep, and enhancing protective factors, such as positive affect and optimism, can have beneficial effects on chronic pain and pain-related outcomes.

- Optimal management for clinicians treating patients with chronic pain is based on targeting the underlying mechanisms of pain and tailoring the management modality using a multimodal approach.

DISCLOSURE

D. Minhas has no disclosures. D.J. Clauw has performed consulting for Pfizer, Lilly, Aptinyx, Zynerba, Lundbeck, Tonix, and Samumed and has received research funds from Aptinyx and Lundbeck.

REFERENCES

1. Stanos S, Brodsky M, Argoff C, et al. Rethinking chronic pain in a primary care setting. Postgrad Med 2016;128(5):502–15.
2. Ablin JN, Cohen H, Neumann L, et al. Coping styles in fibromyalgia: effect of comorbid posttraumatic stress disorder. Rheumatol Int 2008;28(7):649–56.
3. Kidd BL, Urban LA. Mechanisms of inflammatory pain. Br J Anaesth 2001; 87(1):3–11.

4. Basbaum AI, Bautista DM, Scherrer G, et al. Cellular and molecular mechanisms of pain. Cell 2009;139(2):267–84.
5. Pinho-Ribeiro FA, Verri WA Jr, Chiu IM. Nociceptor Sensory Neuron-Immune Interactions in Pain and Inflammation. Trends Immunol 2017;38(1):5–19.
6. Woolf CJ, Salter MW. Neuronal plasticity: increasing the gain in pain. Science 2000;288(5472):1765–9.
7. Coderre TJ, Katz J, Vaccarino AL, et al. Contribution of central neuroplasticity to pathological pain: Review of clinical and experimental evidence. Pain 1993;52(3):259–85.
8. Schaible HG, Grubb BD. Afferent and spinal mechanisms of joint pain. Pain 1993;55(1):5–54.
9. Kosek E, Cohen M, Baron R, et al. Do we need a third mechanistic descriptor for chronic pain states? Pain 2016;157(7):1382–6.
10. McDermid AJ, Rollman GB, McCain GA. Generalized hypervigilance in fibromyalgia: Evidence of perceptual amplification. Pain 1996;66(2–3):133–44.
11. Freynhagen R, Baron R, Gockel U, et al. painDETECT: a new screening questionnaire to identify neuropathic components in patients with back pain. Curr Med Res Opin 2006;22(10):1911–20.
12. Veasley CCD, Clauw DJ, Cowley T, et al. Impact of chronic overlapping pain conditions on public health and the urgent need for safe and effective treatment: 2015 analysis and policy recommendations. Chronic Pain Research Alliance. 2015. Available at: http://wwwchronicpainresearch.org/public/CPRA_WhitePaper_2015-FINAL-Digitalpdf.
13. Woolf CJ. Central sensitization: implications for the diagnosis and treatment of pain. Pain 2011;152(3 Suppl):S2–15.
14. Wolfe F. Fibromyalgianess. In:2009.
15. Winthrop KL, Weinblatt ME, Bathon J, et al. Unmet need in rheumatology: Reports from the Targeted Therapies meeting 2019. In:2020.
16. Basu N, Kaplan CM, Ichesco E, et al. Neurobiologic Features of Fibromyalgia Are Also Present Among Rheumatoid Arthritis Patients. Arthritis Rheumatol 2018;70(7):1000–7.
17. Lee YC, Bingham CO 3rd, Edwards RR, et al. Association between pain sensitization and disease activity in patients with rheumatoid arthritis: a cross-sectional study. Arthritis Care Res (Hoboken) 2018;70(2):197–204.
18. Hawley DJ, Wolfe F. Pain, disability, and pain/disability relationships in seven rheumatic disorders: a study of 1,522 patients. J Rheumatol 1991;18(10):1552–7.
19. Grygiel-Gorniak B, Limphaibool N, Puszczewicz M. Cytokine secretion and the risk of depression development in patients with connective tissue diseases. Psychiatry Clin Neurosci 2019;73(6):302–16.
20. Asmundson GJ, Katz J. Understanding the co-occurrence of anxiety disorders and chronic pain: state-of-the-art. Depress Anxiety 2009;26(10):888–901.
21. Meints SM, Edwards RR. Evaluating psychosocial contributions to chronic pain outcomes. Prog Neuropsychopharmacol Biol Psychiatry 2018;87(Pt B):168–82.
22. Cimmino MA, Ferrone C, Cutolo M. Epidemiology of chronic musculoskeletal pain. Best Pract Res Clin Rheumatol 2011;25(2):173–83.
23. Afari N, Ahumada SM, Wright LJ, et al. Psychological trauma and functional somatic syndromes: a systematic review and meta-analysis. Psychosom Med 2014;76(1):2–11.
24. Harte SE, Harris RE, Clauw DJ. The neurobiology of central sensitization. J Appl Biobehavioral Res 2018;23(2).

25. Jones CP. Levels of racism: a theoretic framework and a gardener's tale. Am J Public Health 2000;90(8):1212–5.

26. Walker Taylor JL, Campbell CM, Thorpe RJ Jr, et al. Pain, racial discrimination, and depressive symptoms among african american women. Pain Manag Nurs 2018;19(1):79–87.

27. Choy EH. The role of sleep in pain and fibromyalgia. Nat Rev Rheumatol 2015; 11(9):513–20.

28. Hassett AL, Finan PH. The role of resilience in the clinical management of chronic pain. Curr Pain Headache Rep 2016;20(6):39.

29. Bird HA, Dixon JS. The measurement of pain. Baillieres Clin Rheumatol 1987;1(1): 71–89.

30. Ablin K, Clauw DJ. From fibrositis to functional somatic syndromes to a bell-shaped curve of pain and sensory sensitivity: evolution of a clinical construct. Rheum Dis Clin North Am 2009;35(2):233–51.

31. Williams DA, Clauw DJ. Understanding fibromyalgia: lessons from the broader pain research community. J Pain 2009;10(8):777–91.

32. Diatchenko L, Nackley AG, Slade GD, et al. Catechol-O-methyltransferase gene polymorphisms are associated with multiple pain-evoking stimuli. Pain 2006; 125(3):216–24.

33. Lee YC, Lu B, Edwards RR, et al. The role of sleep problems in central pain processing in rheumatoid arthritis. Arthritis Rheum 2013;65(1):59–68.

34. Graven-Nielsen T, Arendt-Nielsen L. Assessment of mechanisms in localized and widespread musculoskeletal pain. Nat Rev Rheumatol 2010;6(10):599–606.

35. Joharatnam N, McWilliams DF, Wilson D, et al. A cross-sectional study of pain sensitivity, disease-activity assessment, mental health, and fibromyalgia status in rheumatoid arthritis. Arthritis Res Ther 2015;17:11.

36. Tracey I, Mantyh PW. The cerebral signature for pain perception and its modulation. Neuron 2007;55(3):377–91.

37. Buckner RL, Andrews-Hanna JR, Schacter DL. The brain's default network: anatomy, function, and relevance to disease. Ann N Y Acad Sci 2008;1124:1–38.

38. Napadow V, Kim J, Clauw DJ, et al. Decreased intrinsic brain connectivity is associated with reduced clinical pain in fibromyalgia. Arthritis Rheum 2012;64(7): 2398–403.

39. Gracely RH, Petzke F, Wolf JM, et al. Functional magnetic resonance imaging evidence of augmented pain processing in fibromyalgia. Arthritis Rheum 2002; 46(5):1333–43.

40. Cook DB, Lange G, Ciccone DS, et al. Functional imaging of pain in patients with primary fibromyalgia. J Rheumatol 2004;31(2):364–78.

41. Jensen KB, Loitoile R, Kosek E, et al. Patients with fibromyalgia display less functional connectivity in the brain's pain inhibitory network. Mol Pain 2012;8:32.

42. Lopez-Sola M, Pujol J, Wager TD, et al. Altered functional magnetic resonance imaging responses to nonpainful sensory stimulation in fibromyalgia patients. Arthritis Rheumatol 2014;66(11):3200–9.

43. Lopez-Sola M, Woo CW, Pujol J, et al. Towards a neurophysiological signature for fibromyalgia. Pain 2017;158(1):34–47.

44. Harris RE. Elevated excitatory neurotransmitter levels in the fibromyalgia brain. Arthritis Res Ther 2010;12(5):141.

45. Harris RE, Napadow V, Huggins JP, et al. Pregabalin rectifies aberrant brain chemistry, connectivity, and functional response in chronic pain patients. Anesthesiology 2013;119(6):1453–64.

46. Foerster BR, Petrou M, Edden RA, et al. Reduced insular gamma-aminobutyric acid in fibromyalgia. Arthritis Rheum 2012;64(2):579–83.

47. Harper DE, Ichesco E, Schrepf A, et al. Relationships between brain metabolite levels, functional connectivity, and negative mood in urologic chronic pelvic pain syndrome patients compared to controls: A MAPP research network study. Neuroimage Clin 2018;17:570–8.

48. Russell IJ, Holman AJ, Swick TJ, et al. Sodium oxybate reduces pain, fatigue, and sleep disturbance and improves functionality in fibromyalgia: results from a 14-week, randomized, double-blind, placebo-controlled study. Pain 2011;152(5):1007–17.

49. Scott JR, Hassett AL, Schrepf AD, et al. Moderate alcohol consumption is associated with reduced pain and fibromyalgia symptoms in chronic pain patients. Pain Med 2018;19(12):2515–27.

50. Kim CH, Vincent A, Clauw DJ, et al. Association between alcohol consumption and symptom severity and quality of life in patients with fibromyalgia. Arthritis Res Ther 2013;15(2):R42.

51. Harris RE, Clauw DJ, Scott DJ, et al. Decreased central mu-opioid receptor availability in fibromyalgia. J Neurosci 2007;27(37):10000–6.

52. Albrecht DS, Forsberg A, Sandstrom A, et al. Brain glial activation in fibromyalgia - A multi-site positron emission tomography investigation. Brain Behav Immun 2019;75:72–83.

53. Berna C, Leknes S, Holmes EA, et al. Induction of depressed mood disrupts emotion regulation neurocircuitry and enhances pain unpleasantness. Biol Psychiatry 2010;67(11):1083–90.

54. Hess A, Axmann R, Rech J, et al. Blockade of TNF-alpha rapidly inhibits pain responses in the central nervous system. Proc Natl Acad Sci U S A 2011;108(9):3731–6.

55. Rech J, Hess A, Finzel S, et al. Association of brain functional magnetic resonance activity with response to tumor necrosis factor inhibition in rheumatoid arthritis. Arthritis Rheum 2013;65(2):325–33.

56. Schweinhardt P, Kalk N, Wartolowska K, et al. Investigation into the neural correlates of emotional augmentation of clinical pain. Neuroimage 2008;40(2):759–66.

57. Diatchenko L, Fillingim RB, Smith SB, et al. The phenotypic and genetic signatures of common musculoskeletal pain conditions. Nat Rev Rheumatol 2013;9(6):340–50.

58. Nackley AG, Tan KS, Fecho K, et al. Catechol-O-methyltransferase inhibition increases pain sensitivity through activation of both beta2- and beta3-adrenergic receptors. Pain 2007;128(3):199–208.

59. D'Agnelli S, Arendt-Nielsen L, Gerra MC, et al. Fibromyalgia: Genetics and epigenetics insights may provide the basis for the development of diagnostic biomarkers. Mol Pain 2019;15. 1744806918819944.

60. Ciampi de Andrade D, Maschietto M, Galhardoni R, et al. Epigenetics insights into chronic pain: DNA hypomethylation in fibromyalgia-a controlled pilot-study. Pain 2017;158(8):1473–80.

61. Descalzi G, Ikegami D, Ushijima T, et al. Epigenetic mechanisms of chronic pain. Trends Neurosci 2015;38(4):237–46.

62. Clauw DJ, Crofford LJ. Chronic widespread pain and fibromyalgia: what we know, and what we need to know. Best Pract Res Clin Rheumatol 2003;17(4):685–701.

63. McLean SA, Williams DA, Stein PK, et al. Cerebrospinal fluid corticotropin-releasing factor concentration is associated with pain but not fatigue symptoms in patients with fibromyalgia. Neuropsychopharmacology 2006;31(12):2776–82.

64. Gur A, Oktayoglu P. Status of immune mediators in fibromyalgia. Curr Pain Headache Rep 2008;12(3):175–81.
65. Boettger MK, Hensellek S, Richter F, et al. Antinociceptive effects of tumor necrosis factor alpha neutralization in a rat model of antigen-induced arthritis: evidence of a neuronal target. Arthritis Rheum 2008;58(8):2368–78.
66. Obreja O, Biasio W, Andratsch M, et al. Fast modulation of heat-activated ionic current by proinflammatory interleukin 6 in rat sensory neurons. Brain 2005; 128(Pt 7):1634–41.
67. Bazzichi L, Rossi A, Massimetti G, et al. Cytokine patterns in fibromyalgia and their correlation with clinical manifestations. Clin Exp Rheumatol 2007;25(2): 225–30.
68. Caro XJ, Winter EF. The role and importance of small fiber neuropathy in fibromyalgia pain. Curr Pain Headache Rep 2015;19(12):55.
69. Doppler K, Rittner HL, Deckart M, et al. Reduced dermal nerve fiber diameter in skin biopsies of patients with fibromyalgia. Pain 2015;156(11):2319–25.
70. Kim SH, Kim DH, Oh DH, et al. Characteristic electron microscopic findings in the skin of patients with fibromyalgia–preliminary study. Clin Rheumatol 2008;27(3): 407–11.
71. Levine TD, Saperstein DS. Routine use of punch biopsy to diagnose small fiber neuropathy in fibromyalgia patients. Clin Rheumatol 2015;34(3):413–7.
72. Clauw DJ. What is the meaning of "small fiber neuropathy" in fibromyalgia? Pain 2015;156(11):2115 6.
73. Harte SE, Clauw DJ, Hayes JM, et al. Reduced intraepidermal nerve fiber density after a sustained increase in insular glutamate: a proof-of-concept study examining the pathogenesis of small fiber pathology in fibromyalgia. Pain Rep 2017; 2(3):e590.
74. Taylor P, Manger B, Alvaro-Gracia J, et al. Patient perceptions concerning pain management in the treatment of rheumatoid arthritis. J Int Med Res 2010;38(4): 1213–24.
75. Wolfe F, Michaud K, Busch RE, et al. Polysymptomatic distress in patients with rheumatoid arthritis: understanding disproportionate response and its spectrum. Arthritis Care Res (Hoboken) 2014;66(10):1465–71.

Low Back Pain in Adolescent and Geriatric Populations

David G. Borenstein, MD[a],*, Federico Balagué, MD[b]

KEYWORDS

- Adolescent • Geriatric • Scoliosis • Low back pain • Spinal stenosis

KEY POINTS

- Adolescents have back pain in increasing numbers as they grow older.
- Back pain unassociated with a specific cause is the most common diagnosis associated with adolescents.
- Lumbar spinal stenosis is becoming an increasingly frequent clinical problem as the number of geriatric individuals increases.
- Consensus exists in regard to historical factors associated with the diagnosis of lumbar spinal stenosis.
- Debate remains concerning the long-term improved outcome of lumbar spinal stenosis patients treated with surgical decompression versus nonsurgical interventions.

INTRODUCTION

As discussed in the American College of Rheumatology Pain Management Task Force report in 2010, pain is the most common symptom of patients with rheumatic disorders.[1] Both acute pain and chronic pain are associated with inflammatory and noninflammatory rheumatic conditions. The generation of this symptom in the spine may have different origins depending on the underlying disorder (**Table 1**). With such a broad range of disorders, all age groups are at risk. Adolescents and older individuals are the subjects of this article.

ACUTE AND CHRONIC PAIN

Acute spinal pain may be generated by most anatomic structures of the spine except the interior of intervertebral discs. Acute injury to tissues results in a local inflammatory process that is recognized by nociceptive peripheral nerves. When peripheral nerves are damaged, a neuropathic component of pain may become manifest. When pain persists with modification of the pain pathways, uncoupled from the signs of injury

[a] Department of Medicine, The George Washington University Medical Center, Arthritis and Rheumatism Associates, 2021 K Street, Northwest Suite 300, Washington, DC 20006, USA;
[b] Rheumatology Department, HFR Fribourg-hôpital Cantonal, Fribourg 1708, Switzerland
* Corresponding author. Arthritis and Rheumatism Associates, 2021 K Street, Northwest Suite 300, Washington DC 20006.
E-mail address: dborenstein715@aol.com

Rheum Dis Clin N Am 47 (2021) 149–163
https://doi.org/10.1016/j.rdc.2020.12.001
0889-857X/21/© 2020 Elsevier Inc. All rights reserved.

Table 1	
Disorders associated with low back pain	
Mechanical	*Rheumatologic*
Muscle strain	Ankylosing spondylitis
Herniated intervertebral disk	Reactive arthritis
OA	Psoriatic arthritis
Spinal stenosis	Enteropathic arthritis
Spondylolisthesis	Diffuse idiopathic skeletal hyperostosis
Adolescent/adult scoliosis	Fibromyalgia
Infectious	Polymyalgia rheumatica
Osteomyelitis	*Endocrinologic*
Discitis	Osteomalacia
Pyogenic sacroiliitis	Osteoporosis
Herpes zoster	Parathyroid disease
Neoplastic/infiltrative	Microcrystalline disease
Osteoid osteoma	*Referred pain*
Osteoblastoma	Aortic aneurysm
Osteochondroma	Pancreatitis
Giant cell tumor	Gall bladder disease
Gaucher disease	Kidney
Skeletal metastases	Bladder
Multiple myeloma	Uterus
Chordoma	Ovary
Neurologic/psychiatric	Prostate
Neuropathic arthropathy	*Miscellaneous*
Neuropathies	Paget disease
Psychogenic rheumatism	Vertebral sarcoidosis
Malingering	Retroperitoneal fibrosis
	Subacute bacterial endocarditis

Modified from Borenstein DG, Wiesel SW, Boden SD. Low Back and Neck Pain: Comprehensive Diagnosis and Management, 3rd edition Appendix A Philadelphia: WB Saunders 2004. p. 870 to 889; with permission.

and inflammation, acute pain becomes chronic and a problem unto itself.[2] Under these circumstances, changes in the central nervous system, such as central sensitization and increased psychological response to pain, make treatment of the disorder more difficult. In both adolescents and geriatric patients, peripheral, neuropathic, and central components of pain may be playing roles in their complaints. These considerations are important when prescribing nonpharmacologic and pharmacologic therapies for these patients.[3]

ADOLESCENT SPINE DISORDERS
Epidemiology

Low back pain (LBP) affects upwards of 80% of the world's population. The common cold is the only disorder that occurs more frequently than spinal pain. The incidence of LBP in the United States is estimated at 59 million individuals in a 3-month period.[4]

In regard to adolescents, a cross-sectional survey of 3669 healthy individuals 10 years to 18 years of age demonstrated that 33% reported back pain in the previous year. Of these, 26.3% reported severe pain (defined as pain intensity $\geq$7 on a 0–10 scale). The prevalence increased with age and was above 45% in the 17-year and 18-year age groups. Pain was located most often in the lumbar region (68.9%) followed by the thoracic, sacral, and cervical regions.[5] In this same cohort, 40.9% of adolescents with back pain received some form of treatment, including physical therapy (most frequently, massage chiropractic adjustments) or medication.

A Danish birth cohort study, including 46,726 children, using a definition of pain combining both frequency and intensity of pain, reported that 14.1% of the participants had severe (3.7%) or moderate (10.4%) pain. For both categories, girls reported more LBP than boys. In terms of impact, approximately 6% of the cohort reported greater than 2-times daily-life consequences by means of a composite measure based on questions about school absenteeism, physical activity restrictions, and health care utilization.[6]

Overall, children and adolescents seem to tolerate back pain better than their adult counterparts but quality of life (QOL) is reduced in subjects reporting multiple painful regions[7] or whole-body pain.[8]

Adolescents self-reporting LBP and whole-body pain showed a decreased QOL but also had more health problems (unrelated to the spine) and more life events (unrelated to health) than adolescents who were free of pain or those who reported pain limited to the lower back.[8]

Causes

Psychological factors are stronger predictors of incident LBP than mechanical factors in adolescent populations. In these individuals, an organic etiology for back pain cannot be found despite thorough investigation. A large study analyzed the data of 215,592 American adolescents presenting with LBP from 2007 to 2010. During 1 year after the initial presentation, patients were tracked for imaging obtained and eventual subsequent spinal pathology diagnoses. More than 80% of patients had no identifiable diagnosis at follow-up.[9] Family structure also may play a role in the frequency of back pain as a complaint. The frequency of a weekly complaint of back pain in male adolescents ranged from 8.5% among boys with joint physical custody to 15.5% in single-parent paternal homes. Among female adolescents, the values ranged from 19.1% in girls living in a nuclear family to 28.4% for those in a step family.[10]

As with older adults, mechanical disorders do cause LBP in adolescents.[11] A spectrum of these disorders, as listed in **Table 2**, include muscle strain, disk herniation, spondylolysis, spondylolisthesis, Scheuermann disease, and scoliosis.

Early-onset scoliosis is defined as lateral curvature of the spine greater than 10° with onset before the age of 10 years. The category includes several types: congenital (i.e., structural abnormalities of the spine or thorax), neuromuscular, miscellaneous (i.e. any other syndrome excluding the previous 2 types), and idiopathic. In terms of age, scoliosis is named infantile (ie, onset from birth to 2 years of age), juvenile (ie, onset from 3 years to 9 years of age), or adolescent (ie, onset from 10 years to 18 years). Most adolescents with nonprogressive idiopathic scoliosis can be seen by a primary care physician or rheumatologist and do not require active treatment.[19] Characteristics of adolescent scoliosis are listed in **Box 1**.

Inflammatory illnesses, including spondyloarthritis, discitis, tumors (both benign and malignant), and neurologic neoplasms occur less frequently than mechanical disorders.[23]

Table 2
Adolescent low back pain studies

Reference	Study Design	Study Population	Study Findings	Comments
Ramirez et al,[12] 2019	Retrospective LBP patients with whole-spine MRI Patients with spondylolysis excluded	N = 388 Women—270 Men—118 Age 10–18 y	158 abnormal MRI Disk disease 122 Syringomyelia 4 Spinal cord tumor 4 Tethered cord 2 Paraspinal cystic mass 2 Bone edema 1	Incidental findings —Schmorl nodes Ovarian/renal cysts Hemangiomas Liver mass Facet joint disease
Yamashita et al,[13] 2019	Retrospective LBP athletes—diagnosis by GO vs SS	N = 69 Women—15 Men—54 Age 9–19 y (15.2 y ± 2.3 y)	GO vs SS Lysis 47 vs 51 Disk[a] 7 vs 11 Facet arthritis 1 vs 4 Apophyseal ring Fx 1 vs 1 Unidentified 13 vs 1 Articular process Fx 0 vs 1	SS provided a second opinion to patients—ordered more STIR-MRIs and functional blocks than GO
Brooks et al,[14] 2018	Retrospective Birth to 18 y old Pediatric emergency room Back pain chief complaint 1-year period	N = 232 encounters 177 study subjects Women—103 Men—74 Age <4 y—2.8%; 4–12 y—37.9%; >12 y—59.3%	Discharge diagnoses Nonspecific LBP—76.8% Other noninfectious 12.4% Other infectious 8.5% Radiology performed 37.9% Abnormal findings 16.9% Laboratory tests 35%	Plain radiographs—not CT or MRI associated with pathology 21% had problems unrelated to spine (abdominal, GU, GYN)
Yang et al,[9] 2017	Retrospective National insurance database 2007–2010 Consults for LBP Followed for 1 y	N = 215,592 Women—57% Men—43% Age 10–14 y—35% Age 15–19 y—65%	Database diagnosis LBP unspecified—80.3% Spasm—8.9% Scoliosis—4.7% Degenerative disk—1.7% Disk herniation—1.3% Spondylolysis, olisthesis, infection, tumor, fracture <1%	84%—no imaging

Study	Design/Setting	Demographics	Findings	Comments
MacDonald et al,[15] 2016	Retrospective Pediatric sports clinic 242 encounters (71 initial) 1-y duration	N = 93 Women—50 Men—43 Age 14.1 y ± 2.3 y	Nonspecific LBP 148 Scoliosis 17 The numbers refer to visits.	Micheli Functional Scale Validation study Positive correlation Oswestry Disability Index
Gennari et al,[16] 2015	Retrospective Single-center 2009–2014	N = 116 (LBP in 69) Age 13.6 y Tumors and dysraphism excluded	Nonspecific LBP 32 Scoliosis 31 Scheuermann 23 Spondylolysis 13 Spondylolisthesis 5 Osteoid osteoma 1 Eosinophilic granuloma 1	Low numbers for a 5-y study
Ramirez et al,[17] 2015	Prospective Single-center 2 y duration Systematic approach to chief complaint—LBP	N = 261 (8.6% of all visits) Women—177 Men—84 Age 4-18 y, mean age 13.9 y Diagnostics yield with history, physical examination, plain radiographs (8.8%); bone scan (22%); MRI (36%)	34% identifiable pathology Scoliosis—90 (Cobb angle >25° in 20 patients)	Scoliosis not included as a source of pain
Miller et al,[18] 2013	Retrospective 8-y duration	N = 2846 Women—63% Men—37% Mean age 14.3 y	Nonspecific LBP 2159 Spondylolysis 136 Spondylolisthesis 59	No mention of scoliosis

Abbreviations: FX, fracture; GO, general orthopedists; GU, genitourinary; GYN, gynecologic; SS, spine surgeons; STIR, short tau inversion recovery.
[a] In the article by Yamashita and colleagues, the numbers of disk herniation and discogenic pain are presented separately. The 2 categories have been pooled together in this table.

> **Box 1**
> **Characteristics of adolescent scoliosis**
>
> 1. Adolescent scoliosis has onset at age greater than 10 years and less than 18 years.[20]
> 2. In terms of etiology, a vast majority of cases are idiopathic (adolescent idiopathic scoliosis).
> 3. The overall prevalence ranges from 0.47% to 5.2%.
> 4. Taking into account the prevalence of backache in adolescents (general population), back pain is NOT frequently a relevant problem in teenagers with adolescent idiopathic scoliosis.
> 5. The previous statement does NOT apply to scoliotic adults who frequently report significant back pain secondary to degenerative changes in the spine.
> 6. Adolescents' back pain correlates better with patients' self-perception of their image than with number of abnormal spinal biomechanical variables.
> 7. Pain catastrophizing has been reported to be an important construct in adolescent idiopathic scoliosis–related pain and should be evaluated.[21]
> 8. Skeletally mature patients with curves less than 40°–45° should be observed if there is no pain, no progression, and no imbalance.[22]
> 9. The main predictors of outcome are the magnitude of the curve (Cobb angle), the stage of skeletal maturity (different methods of evaluation exist), and the remaining growth potential.

Clinical Evaluation

History/physical examination

As with adults, characteristics of the onset, quality, duration, location, and radiation of pain may be helpful identifying an underlying pathology. For example, for pain radiating to the groin, particularly in a female adolescent, unrecognized hip dysplasia may be the cause.

A study attempted to determine the sensitivity, specificity, and likelihood ratios of constant pain, night pain, and abnormal neurologic examination to predict the presence of an underlying positive finding (based on magnetic resonance imaging [MRI]) as a cause of back pain. In this series, 388 patients (mean age 14.5 years ± 2.6 years) underwent MRI, which showed any pathologic condition in 158 (40.8%). Of these, 122 (31.4% of the whole sample) presented disk disease, 3.6% had other pathologic findings, and 5.8% had findings considered incidental. An abnormal neurologic examination (in only 2% of cases) appeared to be the strongest predictor for the presence of any underlying pathologic condition, with very low sensitivity (0.05) and good specificity (0.95).[12]

Imaging

Plain radiographs remain the best screening examination for adolescents with back pain. The anteroposterior view demonstrates vertebral body alignment. Lateral view reveals disk space narrowing, end-plate irregularities, and bony modifications. Oblique views are not needed because spondylolysis is identified on the anteroposterior and/or lateral view.[18]

As with adults, MRI identifies anatomic abnormalities in asymptomatic adolescents. Asymptomatic pediatric subjects examined by MRI show frequent incidental findings, mainly disk related. The prevalence of different findings ranges from 2.9% for disk herniation or protrusion to 51.6% for abnormal nucleus shape. Degenerative disk disease occurs in 19.6% and disk space narrowing in 33.7%.[24]

A systematic review and meta-analysis reported the prevalence rates in nonathletes without LBP, in athletes with LBP, and in athletes without LBP. The pooled prevalence rates were, respectively, 22%, 44%, and 22% for disk degeneration; 1%, 38%, and 13% for herniated discs; 5%, 22%, and 11% for end-plate changes; and 0%, 30%, and 6% for pars fractures.[25]

Feldman and colleagues[26] evaluated their algorithmic approach on a group of 87 adolescents (mean age 13.4 years). Specific diagnoses were obtained in 21 cases with initial radiographs. Of the 66 subjects with negative radiographic findings, MRI was obtained in 19 cases of patients who reported having constant pain, night pain, or radicular pain and/or who had an abnormality on neurologic examination. Ten of the 19 patients had MRI findings that were positive for a specific diagnosis. Overall, of 31 patients with a specific diagnosis, radiographs already showed the pathology in 21 cases whereas MRI was necessary in 10 additional cases. The usefulness of the main clinical variables were summarized as follows: sensitivity ranged from 15% (for thoracic pain) to 67% (lumbar pain), specificity from 54% (lumbar pain) to 100% (radicular pain or abnormal neurologic examination), positive predictive value from 17% (thoracic pain) to 100% (radicular pain or abnormal neurologic examination), and negative predictive value from 56% (thoracic pain) to 75% (lumbar pain).[26] In a French cohort of 116 adolescents evaluated over a 5-year period, the largest group was 32 individuals with a diagnosis of nonspecific LBP. The other groups included 31 with scoliosis, 23 with Scheuermann disease, 13 with spondylolysis, 5 with spondylolisthesis, 8 with transitional vertebral abnormalities, 2 with disk herniations, 1 with osteoid osteoma, and 1 with eosinophilic granuloma.[16]

Management

Most of the published series of adolescent patients show a majority of individuals have mechanical causes for LBP and consequently a majority are treated conservatively.[11] Nonsurgical therapy may include activity modification for a period of rest. Nonsteroidal anti-inflammatory agents may be useful. For children with more chronic symptoms, core strengthening and improved flexibility are helpful. Exercise treatment has been found effective in 4 studies for the treatment of LBP, with an average improvement of almost 3 on a pain visual analog scale over the previous month, but has no effect of reducing the prevalence of LBP in adolescents.[27]

The use of opioids for therapy for LBP and chronic pain in general remains controversial. A Cochrane systematic review has highlighted the complete absence of studies eligible for the review, preventing the investigators from commenting about the efficacy or harm of opioids in adolescents.[28] The need for more research has been highlighted in a study of effect the impact of prescription opioids had on 140 of the 283 patients aged 18 years to 23 years followed at a tertiary-care pain clinic[29] The impact of pain-related interference with activities of daily living along with the use of opioid drugs impeded the expected transition to young adulthood with age-appropriate development of cognition, emotion, behavior, and stress responses needed to cope with a chronic condition.

A determination in regard to nonsurgical or surgical therapy depends on the natural history of the malady and its potential impact on adult QOL. The aim of treatment is to resolve pain in adolescence, if possible, to forego the chronicity of the process as an adult.[29]

Health Care Transition

The transition from pediatric, parent-supervised health care to more independent, patient-centered adult care is not an automatic process.[30] Adult rheumatologists must be aware that this transition may be difficult for an adolescent with a chronic condition like LBP. A vast majority of US adolescents do not receive any transition preparation. A major barrier, for example, is difficulty in leaving their pediatric clinician with whom they have had a long-standing relationship. Communication between the pediatric and adult rheumatologists can help bridge the transition of care.

Summary—Adolescent Spine Disorders

The prevalence of LBP increases with age from childhood and approaches the values found in adults by the end of adolescence. Specific diagnoses are identified more frequently in juveniles than in adults, but nonspecific LBP remains the most frequent diagnosis in adolescents. Combining an extensive clinical evaluation and imaging studies leads to the identification of an increased number of spinal pathologies. Nevertheless, the results of imaging studies in asymptomatic subjects show an important number of incidental findings. Adolescents with nonspecific LBP usually can be managed with some form of nonsurgical therapy, including exercise.

GERIATRIC SPINE DISORDERS (SPINAL STENOSIS)
Epidemiology

In 2010, a Global Burden of Disease study ranked LBP the highest of the 291 conditions studied in terms of years lost to disability.[31] In 2015, an update to that study estimated that 266 million individuals (3.63%) worldwide had lumbar degenerative spine disease.[32] Based on population sizes, low-income and middle-income countries had 4-times as many cases as high-income countries; 39 million individuals (0.53%) worldwide had spondylolisthesis, 403 million (5.5%) individuals had symptomatic disk degeneration, and 103 million (1.41%) had spinal stenosis annually.

Cause

The first manifestations of aging in the spine occur in the intervertebral discs. The nucleus pulposus loses its resistance to compressive forces and the annulus fibrosus fissures, resulting in degeneration of fibers. With an inadequate annulus fibrosus, the nucleus pulposus protrudes or herniates. The result of this process is an intervertebral disk that is narrower at that interspace.

Secondary to disk space narrowing, increased pressure is placed on apophyseal joint cartilage. The severity of facet joint osteoarthritis (OA) is related directly to the degree of disk space narrowing. The converse does not occur, so disk degeneration is the initiating factor in facet arthritis.[33] The resulting biomechanical insufficiency from disk degeneration, including loss of paraspinous muscle mass, transfers forces posteriorly to the ligaments and facet joints. Disk degeneration affects women and men equally and increases with age. Like other osteoarthritic joints in the body, the presence of modification of joint anatomy is not related directly to the presence of pain.[34] Localized back pain occurs when alterations in facet joint alignment and pressure results in articular pain.

In an attempt to decrease pressure on painful joints, the lumbar lordosis may flatten. Placing pressure on the anterior components of the vertebrae decompresses the facet joints but places increasing tension in the supporting muscles, which may fatigue and become painful.

The growth of facet osteophytes, protrusion of intervertebral discs, and redundancy of the ligamentum flavum reduce the space in the spinal canal or neural foramen. With decreased volume, the vasa nervorum is compressed. With decreased blood flow, neurogenic claudication occurs with associated pain in the corresponding nerve distribution. With reversal of the compression, blood flow is restored and pain is relieved. The longer the duration of the vascular compromise, the more persistent and total becomes the neural dysfunction. The clinical correlate of this pathophysiology is radicular pain followed by numbness and muscular weakness in the lower extremities.

Clinical Evaluation

History/physical examination

Neurogenic claudication is the most common symptom associated with lumbar spinal stenosis (LSS). Pain that is associated with standing or walking occurs in the buttock, thigh, or lower leg. The patterns of back pain and/or leg pain vary with the patients with the disorder. Most patients have back pain and leg pain. A smaller proportion of patients have leg pain alone. Some patients have bilateral leg pain. The distribution of leg pain may be different in each extremity. Multiple dermatomes may be affected. In the setting of widespread distribution of symptoms, ascribing compression to a single nerve root lesion is difficult. In addition to pain, patients may have paresthesias, numbness, or weakness. Neurogenic claudication is relieved by flexing at the waist, lying down, or sitting.

A total of 279 musculoskeletal physicians participated in a Delphi method to reach a consensus concerning the historical factors associated most closely with LSS.[35] The most important history items for diagnosis of LSS included leg pain or buttock pain while walking, flexing forward to relieve symptoms, feeling relief when using a shopping cart or bicycle, motor or sensory disturbance while walking, normal and symmetric foot pulses, lower extremity weakness, and LBP. The presence of 6 of these characteristics is associated with an 80% certainty of LSS diagnosis.

LSS and hip OA occur in older individuals. Symptoms and signs of these 2 conditions may overlap. A group of 51 musculoskeletal physicians participated in a series of surveys to differentiate hip OA from LSS.[36] Eight symptoms favoring hip OA over LSS included groin pain, knee pain, pain that decreases with continued walking, pain that occurs immediately with walking, pain that occurs immediately with standing, pain getting in/out of a car, pain with dressing the symptomatic leg, and difficulty reaching the foot of the symptomatic leg while dressing. Three symptoms favoring LSS over hip OA included pain below the knee, leg tingling and/or numbness, and some pain in both legs. Symptoms that did not discriminate included decreased pain with using a shopping cart, back pain, weakness and/or heaviness of a leg, buttock pain, poor balance, increased pain with weight bearing on painful leg, and stair walking.

Patients with LSS may have no findings on physical examination in a seated position. Abnormalities may appear only after stressing a patient with walking until leg pain appears.[37] Sciatica caused by LSS is distinct from radiculopathy associated with an intervertebral disk in that objective neurologic abnormalities like asymmetric reflexes are found in a minority.[38] Also of utility is checking for the presence of foot and ankle pulses to identify those individuals who may be at risk for vascular claudication.

Seven physical findings favoring hip OA over LSS include limited weight bearing on painful leg when standing, observed limping, and pain or restricted motion with 5 hip maneuvers. Neurologic deficits favored a diagnosis of LSS over hip OA.[36]

Imaging

Many radiographic techniques exist to evaluate LSS patients.[39] The least sensitive but most available is plain radiographs of the lumbar spine. Identifiable abnormalities include end-plate sclerosis, disk-narrowing, facet-joint hypertrophy, spondylolisthesis, and neural foraminal osteophytes. Soft tissues and neural elements are not visible. Radiographic abnormalities are compatible, but not diagnostic, of spinal stenosis because similar radiographic abnormalities are noted in asymptomatic individuals. MRI can identify bony anatomy, neural elements, vascular structures, and other soft tissues like ligamentum flavum and paraspinous muscles. MRI is the radiographic technique with the greatest potential for identifying anatomic abnormalities associated with LSS. Specific measurements, however, indicative of a definitive diagnosis of LSS are yet to be determined[40] (**Fig. 1**).

Computed tomography (CT), with or without myelography, is a technique using larger exposure of radiation to identify the osseous structures in the spine. This technique is used when patients are unable to have an MRI because of claustrophobia, pacemakers, or other contraindications to MRI.[41]

Also of note is the lack of benefit of early radiographic evaluation in older adults without radiculopathy with an improved outcome at 1 year.[42] The degree of disability was the same in those who had radiographs (Roentgenograms or MRI) versus those treated without the benefit of imaging.

Diagnosis of LSS remains a clinical one because no specific set of clinical, radiographic, or interventional tests is definitive. Therefore, the patient with LSS is characterized by specific historical and physical findings and confirmed, but not diagnosed, by radiographic techniques documenting the compression of neural structures.

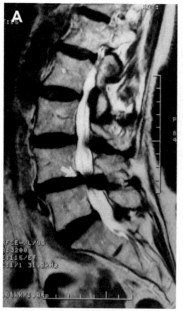
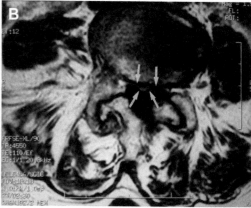

Fig. 1. MRIs of the lumbar spine of a 92-year-old woman with leg numbness and difficulty ambulating. Sagittal (A) and axial (B) views demonstrating severe stenosis at L4-L5 (*arrows*) caused by facet joint osteophytes, a protruding intervertebral disk, and redundant ligamentum flavum. (*From* Borenstein DG, Wiesel SW, Bowden SD. Low Back and Neck Pain: Comprehensive Diagnosis and Management 3rd edition pg. 272; with permission.)

Management

LSS management requires judgment that matches the severity of functional impairment with benefits and risks of interventions. In older adults, determination of their most severe limitation is essential. Is cardiac, pulmonary, or vascular disease their most significant physical limitation? Or is LSS with the development of neurogenic claudication their greatest disability?

The underlying pathophysiology of LSS is the compression of vascular supply to the neural elements. The goal of therapy is to maximize the space in the spinal canal by expanding volume (flexion of the spine) and shrinking inflamed, swollen tissues.

The options include education, weight reduction, exercises, smoking cessation, pharmaceuticals, injections, and surgery. No one therapy works for all patients. A combination of options may be necessary to control symptoms. Surgical decompression is an appropriate choice for individuals who have not responded to nonsurgical interventions or have neurologic compromise that severely impairs function.[43]

Pharmacologic therapies in the forms of nonsteroidal anti-inflammatory medications, acetaminophen, gabapentin, pregabalin, and opioids all have potential toxicities that limit their full potential as therapeutic agents. Duloxetine has an indication for the treatment of chronic LBP but not for the treatment of LSS.[44]

Epidural corticosteroid injections are the most commonly performed outpatient procedures for the treatment of spinal pain.[45] Epidural injections are given in a series of 3. For the pathophysiology of LSS, the injections are delayed until symptoms recur because injections can be given no sooner than every 2 months. The benefits of epidural steroids are time-limited.[46,47]

Surgical decompression is indicated in individuals who have failed medical therapy and are physically incapacitated by spinal stenosis. The goal of surgery is to obtain adequate decompression without causing instability. The difficulty for the spine surgeon is identifying the most symptomatic level and determining the extent of the decompression. The need for fusion and instrumentation remains a controversial decision. It is not clear that individuals who have a fusion necessarily have an improved outcome.[48]

For older adults who are not candidates for decompressive surgery, interspinous spacers are placed with less invasive techniques. The placement of an interspinous spacer in an LSS individual without spondylolisthesis may improve the vertical space in the foramen and decompress the corresponding spinal nerve. Compared with decompressive surgery, spacing devices have fewer complications but higher rates of revision surgery.[49]

Conservative Versus Surgical Treatment

Different studies have followed patients with LSS treated with conservative management versus surgical decompression for variable durations. Some studies have suggested the short-term benefit of decompression whereas long-term follow-up suggests similar outcomes for those treated with either regimen.[43,50,51]

Summary—Geriatric Spine Disorders

The frequency of LSS will increase as a clinical problem as the geriatric population ages. Neurogenic claudication will become a cause of significant disability in those without comorbidities that limit function. Historical factors can help differentiate those patients with LSS from individuals with hip joint arthritis. MRI is the best radiographic technique to reveal those with anatomic findings of nerve compression but is not specific in identifying those who are symptomatic. The aim of therapy is to relieve compression on spinal nerves. Whether surgical decompression or medical therapy is the best method to achieve that end remains to be determined.

CLINICS CARE POINTS

- A systematic, complete, and adapted clinical history and physical examination for adolescents are good guides to the additional investigations needed to choose appropriate management.
- Rheumatologists need to be cognizant of the risks of indiscriminate imaging studies in adolescents that result in overtreatment.
- A critical evaluation of response to therapy is necessary to avoid overlooking specific pathologies that require more aggressive approaches.
- LSS is an increasingly common clinical problem as the population ages.
- Spinal stenosis and hip OA are differentiated with specific historical and physical findings.
- The pros and cons of surgical management have to be weighed carefully in terms of risks and benefits in deciding on appropriate therapy for neurogenic claudication.

DISCLOSURE

D.G. Borenstein, MD—research grant, Abbvie. F. Balagué, MD—the author has nothing to disclose.

REFERENCES

1. American college of rheumatology pain management task force report of the american college of rheumatology pain management task force. Arthritis Care Res 2010;62:590–9.
2. Woller SA, Eddinger KA, Corr M, et al. An overview of pathways encoding nociception. Clin Exp Rheumatol 2017;35(Suppl.107):S40–6.
3. Clauw DJ, Hassett AL. The role of centralized pain in osteoarthritis. Clin Exp Rheumatol 2017;35(Suppl 107):S79–84.
4. Lawrence R, Felson DT, Helmick CG, et al. Estimates of the prevalence of arthritis and other rheumatic conditions in the United States Part II. Arthritis Rheumatol 2008;58:26–35.
5. Fabricant PD, Heath MR, Shachne JM, et al. The epidemiology of back pain in American children and adolescents. Spine (Phila Pa 1976) 2020;45:1135–42.
6. Joergensen AC, Hestbaek L, Andersen PK, et al. Epidemiology of spinal pain in children: a study within the Danish National Birth Cohort. Eur J Pediatr 2019; 178(5):695–706.
7. Goncalves TR, Mediano MFF, Sichieri R, et al. Is health-related quality of life decreased in adolescents with back pain? Spine (Phila Pa 1976) 2018;43(14): E822–9.
8. Balague F, Ferrer M, Rajmil L, et al. Assessing association between low back pain, quality of life, and life events as reported by schoolchildren in a population-based study. Eur J Pediatr 2012;171(3):507–14.
9. Yang S, Werner BC, Singla A, et al. Low back pain in adolescents: a 1-year analysis of eventual diagnoses. J Pediatr Orthop 2017;37(5):344–7.
10. Nilsen SA, Hysing M, Breivik K, et al. Complex families and health complaints among adolescents: a population-based cross-sectional study. Scand J Public Health 2019. https://doi.org/10.1177/1403494819893903.

11. DePaola K, Cuddihy LA. Pediatric spine disorders. Pediatr Clin North Am 2020; 67:185–204.

12. Ramirez N, Olivella G, Valentin P, et al. Are constant pain, night pain, or abnormal neurological examination adequate predictors of the presence of a significant pathology associated with pediatric back pain? J Pediatr Orthop 2019;39(6): e478–81.

13. Yamashita K, Sakai T, Takata Y, et al. Low back pain in adolescent athletes: comparison of diagnoses made by general orthopedic surgeons and spine surgeons. Int J Spine Surg 2019;13(2):178–85.

14. Brooks TM, Friedman LM, Silvis RM, et al. Back pain in a pediatric emergency department: Etiology and evaluation. Pediatr Emerg Care 2018;34(1):e1–6.

15. MacDonald JP, d'Hemecourt PA, Micheli LJ. The reliability and validity of a pediatric back outcome measure. Clin J Sport Med 2016;26(6):490–6.

16. Gennari JM, Themar-Noel C, Panuel M, et al. Adolescent spinal pain: the pediatric orthopedist's point of view. Orthop Traumatol Surg Res 2015;101(6 suppl): S247–50.

17. Ramirez N, Flynn JM, Hill BW, et al. Evaluatiaon of a systematic approach to pediatric back pain: the utility of magnetic resonance imaging. J Pediatr Orthop 2015;35(1):28–32.

18. Miller R, Beck NA, Sampson NR, et al. Imaging modalities for low back pain in children: a review of spondylolysis and undiagnosed mechanical back pain. J Pediatr Orthop 2013;33(3):282–8.

19. Hresko MT. Clinical practice> Idiopahtic scoliosis in adolescents. N Engl J Med 2013;368(9):834–41.

20. Balagué F, Pellisé F. Adolescent idiopathic scoliosis and back pain. Scoliosis Spinal Disord 2016;11(1):27.

21. Teles AR, St-Georges M, Abduljabbar F, et al. Back pain in adolescents with idiopathic scoliosis: the contribution of morphological and psychological factors. Eur Spine J 2020;29(8):1959–71.

22. Agabegi SS, Kazemi N, Sturm PF, et al. Natural history of adolescent idiopathic scoliosis in skeletally mature patients: a critical review. J Am Acad Orthop Surg 2015;12:714–23.

23. Brown J, Lakkol S, Lazenby S, et al. Common neoplastic causes of paediatric and adolescent back pain. Br J Hosp Med 2020;81(5):1–6.

24. Ramadorai U, Hire J, DeVine JG, et al. Incidental findings on magnetic resonance imaging of the spine in the asymptomatic pediatric population: a systematic review. Evid Based Spine Care J 2014;5(2):95–100.

25. Van den Heuvel MM, Oei EHG, Bierma-Zientra SMA, et al. The prevalence of abnormalities in the pediatric spine on MRI: a systematic review and meta-analysis. Spine (Phila Pa 1976) 2020;45(18):e1185–96.

26. Feldman DS, Straight JJ, Badra MI, et al. Evaluation of an algorithmic approach to pediatric back pain. J Pediatr Orthop 2006;26(3):353–7.

27. Michaleff ZA, Kamper SJ, Maher CG, et al. Low back pain in children and adolescents: a systematic review and meta-analysis evaluating the effectiveness of conservative interventions. Eur Spine J 2014;23(10):2046–58.

28. Cooper TE, Fisher E, Gray AL, et al. Opioids for chronic non-cancer pain in children and adolescents. Cochrane Database Syst Rev 2017;7:CD012538.

29. Anastas T, Colpitts K, Ziadni M, et al. Characterizing chronic pain in late adolescence and early adulthood: prescription opioids, marijuana use, obesity, and predictors for greater pain interference. Pain Rep 2018;3(6):e700.

30. White PH, Cooley WC. Transitions clinical report authoring group, American academy of pediatrics, American academy of family physicians, american college of physicians. supporting the health care transition from adolescence to adulthood in the medical home. Pediatrics 2018;142(5):320182587.
31. Hoy D, March L, Brooks P, et al. The global burden of low back pain: estimated from the Global Burden of Disease 2010 study. Ann Rheum Dis 2014;73:968–74.
32. Ravindra VM, Senglaub SS, Rattani A, et al. Degenerative lumbar spine disease: estimating global incidence and worldwide volume. Global Spine J 2018;8(8): 784–94.
33. Butler D, Trafimow JH, Anderson GB, et al. Discs degenerate before facets. Spine (Phila Pa 1976) 1990;15:111–3.
34. Borenstein D. Does osteoarthritis of the lumbar spine cause chronic low back pain? Curr Rheumatol Rep 2004;6:14–9.
35. Tomkins-Lane C, Melloh M, Lurie J, et al. ISSLS Prize Winner: consensus on the clinical diagnosis of lumbar spinal stenosis. Spine (Phila Pa 1976) 2016;41: 1239–46.
36. Rainville J, Bono JV, Laxer EB, et al. Comparison of the history and physical examination for hip osteoarthritis and lumbar spinal stenosis. Spine J 2019;19(6): 1009–18.
37. Johnsson B, Stromqvist B. Symptoms and signs in degeneration of the lumbar spine. J Bone Joint Surg Br 1993;75B:381–5.
38. Katz JN, Dalgas M, Stucki G, et al. Degenerative lumbar spinal stenosis. Diagnostic value of the history and physical examination. Arthritis Rheum 1995;38: 1236–41.
39. Katz JN, HarrisMB. Clinical practice. Lumbar spinal stenosis. N Engl J Med 2008; 358:818–25.
40. De Schepper ET, Overdevest GM, Suri P, et al. Diagnosis of lumbar spinal stenosis. Spine 2013;38(8):E469–81.
41. Kreiner DS, Shaffer WO, Baisden JL, et al. An evidence-based clinical guideline for the diagnosis and treatment of degenerative lumbar spine stenosis (update). Spine J 2013;13:734–43.
42. Jarvik JG, Gold LS, Comstock BA, et al. Association of early imaging for back pain with clinical outcomes in older adults. JAMA 2015;313(11):1143–53.
43. Burgstaller JM, Steurer J, Gravestock I, et al. Long-term results after surgical and nonsurgical treatment in patients with degenerative lumbar spinal stenosis. Spine (Phila Pa 1976) 2020;45:1030–8.
44. Enomoto H, Fujikoshi S, Funai J, et al. Assessment of direct analgesic effect of duloxetine for chronic low back pain: post hoc path analysis of double-blind, placebo-controlled studies. J Pain Res 2017;10:1357–68.
45. Markman JD, Schilling LS. Corticosteroids for pain of spine origin: Epidural and intraarticular administration. Rheum Dis Clin North Am 2016;42:137–55.
46. Fornari M, Robertson SC, Pereira P, et al. Conservative treatment and percutaneous pain relief techniques in patients with lumbar spinal stenosis. WENS Spine Committee recommendations. World Neurosurg 2020;7:100079.
47. Liu K, Liu P, Liu R, et al. Steroid for epidural injection in spinal stenosis: a systematic review and meta-analysis. Drug Des Devel Ther 2015;9:707–16.
48. Forsth P, Olafsson G, Carlsson T, et al. A randomized, controlled trial of fusion surgery for lumbar spinal stenosis. N Engl J Med 2016;374:1413–23.
49. Lafian AM, Torralba KD. Lumbar spinal stenosis in older adults. Rheum Dis Clin North Am 2018;44:501–12.

50. Atlas SJ, Keller RB, Wu YA, et al. Long-term outcomes of surgical and nonsurgical management of lumbar spinal stenosis. Spine (Phila Pa 1976) 2005;30: 927–35.
51. Zaina F, Tomkins-Lane C, Carragee E, et al. Surgical versus non-surgical treatment for lumbar spinal stenosis. Cochrane Database Syst Rev 2016;(1):CD010264.

Basic Mechanisms of Pain in Osteoarthritis

Experimental Observations and New Perspectives

Anne-Marie Malfait, MD, PhD[a],*, Rachel E. Miller, PhD[a], Richard J. Miller, PhD[b]

KEYWORDS

- Osteoarthritis • Pain • Sensitization • DRG neurons • NGF • Innate immunity

KEY POINTS

- Osteoarthritis is one of the primary sources of chronic pain worldwide, representing a major unmet medical need. Current pharmacological interventions do not need patients' needs.
- In the course of progressive osteoarthritis, the nociceptive system of the joint undergoes tremendous anatomical plasticity, as well as changes in the functional properties of neurons.
- The neurotrophin, nerve growth factor (NGF), plays a key role in in these pathogenic processes. Neutralizing antibodies against NGF are in clinical trials for osteoarthritis pain.
- Neuronal pathways are modified by interaction with the degenerating joint tissues they innervate. These extensive cellular interactions provide a substrate for identification of targets for osteoarthritis pain.

INTRODUCTION

Physiologic pain is a protective mechanism that involves the detection of stimuli that have a potentially damaging effect on an organism.[1] Pain-producing noxious stimuli commonly are mechanical, chemical, or thermal in origin and activate the peripheral nerve terminals of specialized sensory neurons that innervate tissues and whose cell bodies are localized in the dorsal root and trigeminal ganglia. These pain-sensing afferents are called nociceptors, and depolarization of their nerve terminals

[a] Department of Internal Medicine, Division of Rheumatology, Rush University Medical Center, Room 714, 1735 W Harrison Street, Chicago, IL 60612, USA; [b] Department of Pharmacology, Northwestern University, Searle Building Room 8-510, 320 E Superior Street, Chicago, IL 60611, USA
* Corresponding author. Division of Rheumatology, Department of Medicine, 1611 West Harrison Street, Suite 510, Chicago, IL 60612.
E-mail address: anne-marie_malfait@rush.edu

Rheum Dis Clin N Am 47 (2021) 165–180
https://doi.org/10.1016/j.rdc.2020.12.002
0889-857X/21/© 2020 Elsevier Inc. All rights reserved.

rheumatic.theclinics.com

initiates the firing of action potentials that invade the dorsal root ganglia (DRG).[2] Studies of the electrophysiologic properties of nociceptors have demonstrated that electrogenesis in these neurons requires the activation of specific types of voltage-gated sodium channels (Na_Vs), $Na_V1.7$, $Na_V1.8$, and $Na_V1.9$. In humans, both gain-of-function and loss-of-function mutations in these genes have been described, and these result in marked pain phenotypes, including congenital insensitivity to pain or erythromelalgia (a rare syndrome characterized by episodes of severe, burning pain, redness, and increased skin temperature, mostly in the feet) among other syndromes (reviewed by Drissi and colleagues[3] and by Emery and coleagues[4]).

The normal processing of pain is altered substantively in response to pathology. In many instances, such as in inflammation or tissue injury, pain pathways become sensitized, so that stimuli that previously were innocuous now trigger painful responses.[2] In some cases, these pain responses become dissociated from their protective functions and ongoing pain is experienced in the absence of physiologically appropriate stimuli. The molecular and cellular mechanisms that mediate pain in association with pathology involve changes to the properties of neurons at all levels of the neuraxis, both in the periphery and in the central nervous system.[2,5]

Osteoarthritis (OA) is one of the major causes of chronic pain in the world.[6] Pain in OA is typically mechanical in nature—for example, patients with knee OA complain that it hurts to climb stairs.[7] In addition to the symptom of pain, OA patients show signs of peripheral and central sensitization, which can be detected by quantitative sensory testing, including reduced pressure pain thresholds and increased temporal summation, both at the OA joint as well as at anatomic sites away from the joint.[8,9] In a majority of patients, OA joint pain is relieved by joint replacement surgery, strongly suggesting that pain signaling in OA continues to be dependent on peripheral triggers throughout the disease process. Mechanistically, this involves the detection of painful stimuli by joint-innervating nociceptors. In mice, chemogenetic methods involving the expression of designer receptors exclusively activated by designer drugs in specific nerve populations can be used to selectively stimulate $G_{i/o}$ protein signaling in order to reduce peripheral sensory nerve activity,[10] and this results in inhibition of pain behaviors in experimental OA models, particularly in early phases of disease.[11,12] On the other hand, acute chemogenetic inhibition of nociceptor function has been reported to be ineffective in ameliorating pain behaviors at late stages of murine experimental OA in 1 study,[11] indicating that other factors that affect pain signaling may be of overriding importance in late-stage disease. This may be important for understanding underlying mechanisms for those patients who experience little pain relief from joint replacement (approximately 20% of patients with knee OA and fewer for hip OA[13]), suggesting that central sensitization in those patients is no longer dependent on peripheral input.[14]

Understanding the mechanisms that underlie OA pain requires, first and foremost, a complete description of the properties of the neuronal pathways that mediate pain signaling in the joint. In the course of chronic progressive disease, these pathways are altered and modified by interaction with the degenerating and remodeling tissues they innervate, and with immune and inflammatory cells that react to the disease.[15-17] The specific changes in the peripheral neuronal pathways underlying joint pain in OA are the focus of this review (For discussion on central mechanisms, readers are referred to other reviews.[8,18,19]) The authors searched PubMed for the following terms: "osteoarthritis", "pain", "sensitization", "DRG neurons", "nociceptors", "mechanosensation", "animal models", "NGF", "DAMPs", and "TLR". First, the sensory nervous system in OA is described, with a focus on recent discoveries, driven by new molecular technologies, such as single-cell RNA sequencing, that are revealing that DRG neurons can be classified into distinct functional classes characterized by expression of selected marker molecules. How these discoveries may be relevant for joint pain in OA are discussed. Then, how the sensory nervous system interacts with its environment in the OA joint and how this modulates pain processing in OA are summarized briefly.

THE NERVOUS SYSTEM IN OSTEOARTHRITIS

It should be realized—and this cannot be stressed too strongly—that because of the chronic nature of OA, the anatomy and physiology of nociception undergo considerable plasticity during the course of the disease. Hence, it is important to understand the pharmacology and physiology of pain as it is manifest during progressive disease rather than in unaffected animals or human subjects. As discussed, the plasticity of the nociceptive system in OA involves changes in the structural, physiologic, and genetic properties of neurons in pain pathways. Understanding the exact nature of this plasticity and how it comes about are key issues if there is to be progress in the treatment of OA-associated pain.

Types of Dorsal Root Ganglia Neurons

Primary sensory afferent neurons, including nociceptors, are pseudo-unipolar in structure, with 1 process attached to the cell body that bifurcates into 2 branches. The peripheral or distal processes of these neurons project to the cutaneous or deep peripheral tissues they innervate, and the other branch, referred to as the proximal process, terminates in the dorsal horn of the spinal cord or sensory nuclei of the brain stem. These sensory neurons are responsible for mediating diverse aspects of somatosensory physiology and are quite heterogeneous anatomically, physiologically, and biochemically. There are clearly distinct types of sensory neurons with different response profiles that underlie their ability to discriminate between different types of sensations, such as heat, cold, pain, and itch, as well as mechanical sensations like touch and proprioception.[20] Numerous investigations have sought to answer the question as to the precise properties of each set of neurons that mediate particular somatosensory functions, including nociception, and how the properties of these neurons change in the face of pathology.

How then is the class of sensory neurons that may mediate OA pain described? The first way that sensory neuron subtypes were categorized was according to their degree of myelination and associated electrophysiological properties, such as conduction velocity. Sensory neurons were shown to be heavily and moderately myelinated Aα and Aβ fibers, thinly myelinated Aδ fibers, and unmyelinated C fibers. The degree of myelination has functional consequences determining the speed of action potential conduction, with heavily myelinated A fibers conducting action potentials the most rapidly.[21] These neurophysiologic differences in conduction velocity also have been associated with discrete functions. Heavily and moderately myelinated A fibers are thought to be generally associated with light touch and proprioception, whereas thinly myelinated Aδ fibers detect innocuous and noxious stimuli. C fibers are unmyelinated and mostly involved in detecting painful stimuli, although some C fibers, termed, *low-threshold mechanoreceptors* (*LTMRs*), also are responsible for relaying innocuous light touch stimulation (such as pleasant touch elicited by the stoking of a soft brush). Nociceptors, the C fibers and Aδ fibers that detect noxious stimuli, can either be polymodal, responding to a variety of noxious stimuli (ie, mechanical and thermal), or unimodal, responding to only a single type of noxious stimulation.[22]

It has become clear, however, that fiber classification alone does not provide a sufficient means of predicting neuronal function.[23] This has led to other complementary methods of sensory neuron classification that depend on the expression of selected marker molecules, such as peptidergic neurotransmitters, ion channels, calcium-binding proteins, and receptors, which indicate some specific function associated with each neuron type. Such markers also allow the identification of sensory neuron types using histologic methods, such as in situ hybridization or immunohistochemistry. From the histologic perspective, large light and the small dark neurons originally were recognized. Large light neurons were shown to stain for neurofilament (NF) 200 and are mostly Aα/β, whereas the small dark neurons are NF 200 negative and mostly correspond to unmyelinated nociceptive C fibers.[24] Additionally, nociceptors can be subdivided based on a limited number of neurochemical features, in particular a division between peptidergic and nonpeptidergic classes, the former being defined by containing neuropeptides, such as substance P and calcitonin gene–related peptide (CGRP), whereas nonpeptidergics traditionally do not contain these neuropeptides but bind the plant lectin Griffonia simplicifolia I-B4 (IB4). The peptidergic neurons are either C-fiber or Aδ-fiber neurons, whereas nonpeptidergic are all are C fibers. Of importance for a discussion of OA pain, it also originally was proposed that a majority of peptidergic neurons express tropomyosin receptor kinase A (TrkA), the high-affinity receptor for the pain-producing neurotrophin, nerve growth factor (NGF), whereas nonpeptidergic neurons do not,[25] although this conclusion may have to be revised based on single-cell RNA sequencing data (discussed later). In recent years, more advanced molecular biology techniques have led to the discovery of an increased number of marker molecules, resulting in the further devolution of these categories into ever more diverse groups. For example, subpopulations of nonpeptidergic neurons express the Mas-related G protein–coupled receptors (Mrgprs), which define at least 2 subgroups of IB4-binding and Ret-expressing nonpeptidergic neurons, MrgprD, MrgprA3/MrgprC11, and MrgprB4.[26] These genetically defined subpopulations also appear functionally relevant, because Mrgprd$^+$ neurons are mechanically responsive,[27] whereas Mrgpra3$^+$ neurons have been linked to response to itch,[28] and Mrgprb4$^+$ neurons appear to play a role in response to light touch of hairy skin.[29]

Although the traditional classification of nociceptors has been an important aid to understanding of pain mechanisms, sensory neuron biology recently has entered the age of microanatomy and function based on the revolutionary use of powerful nucleic sequencing techniques. Single-cell RNA sequencing of large numbers of cells and their transcripts together with bioinformatic procedures enable the unbiased identification of categories of neurons based on their transcriptome profiles.[30,31] These techniques can provide extremely valuable data as to the precise molecular identity of DRG neurons and their specific somatosensory specialization. There is not yet a complete consensus as to the number of DRG neuron classes and their functional specializations, but according to a recent review that parsed the currently published data sets, there may be a total of 18 somatosensory DRG neuron subtypes,[23] which define functional specificity (**Fig. 1**). It also has become clear that all nociceptors, except NP1.1 and NP1.2, can express neuropeptides.[23] Suffice it to say that the precise number of types of DRG neurons and their respective functions are likely to be much greater than originally anticipated. Importantly, these current classifications are based on studies in young adult healthy mice. Now, these advanced molecular and genetic techniques can be used to explore how the molecular and functional identity of DRG neurons is altered during the course of chronic painful diseases, such as OA. Such studies will provide a basis for rational experiments to explore how these different subsets of nociceptors relate to pain in joints affected OA, for example, through functional manipulation of subsets of sensory neurons. It can be expected

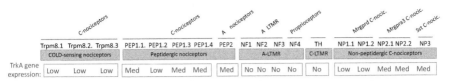

Fig. 1. Classification of DRG sensory neurons, based on Emery and Ernfors.[23] The investigators used http://mousebrain.org/genesearch.html, which shows gene expression throughout the mouse nervous system based on single-cell RNA-seq profiling, to determine *Ntrk1* (TrkA) expression in each subtype. High expression of *Ntrk1* is found in sympathetic neurons, whereas C and Aδ nociceptors show low to medium expression. A-LTMR neurons and TH C-LTMRs do not express *Ntrk1*. NP, nonpeptidergic; nocic., nociceptors; PEP, peptidergic; Sst, somatostatin; TH, tyrosine hydroxylase.

that this will lead to the identification of specific neuronal targets and development of novel targeted analgesic therapies.

Joint Innervation in Osteoarthritis

A critical step in unraveling the contribution of sensory neurons to joint pain in OA is to describe precisely where different relevant subsets of neurons are located in the joint. OA pathology affects all joint tissues, including articular cartilage, subchondral bone, synovium, menisci, and ligaments and many of these tissues are innervated by free nerve endings of nociceptors. In healthy joints, the capsule, ligaments, menisci, periosteum and subchondral bone—but not articular cartilage—all have been shown to be richly innervated by sensory and sympathetic neurons, with a vast majority of sensory afferents being nociceptors.[32–34] It also has emerged that in the course of OA, the innervation may change—for example, anatomic studies in human OA knee joints and in rat models have revealed vascular penetration and nerve growth in the menisci, in osteophytes, and in the subchondral bone.[35,36] Importantly, the appearance of osteochondral channels that breach the tidemark between the subchondral bone and the articular cartilage was described many years ago in human subjects with OA as well as in rat models of OA, with evidence that these channels contain neurons (PGP9.5 staining) and blood vessels.[35,37–39] More recently, Aso and colleagues[39] expanded their work to show that the presence of CGRP-immunoreactive nociceptors in these osteochondral channels was associated with pain in human OA knees as well as in a rat meniscal transection model.

Recent identification of specific molecular markers for different types of DRG neurons, as described previously, enables the selective genetic labeling of these neurons in mice using appropriate Cre-recombinase driver lines to produce the expression of fluorescent markers in selected types of neurons. The resulting mice can be used for examining the precise innervation of the knee joint and whether this is altered during the development of OA in mouse models, something that never has been examined previously. In order to define changes in joint innervation that might contribute to OA pain, Obeidat and colleagues employed fluorescently labeled Na$_V$1.8-expressing neurons to investigate the nociceptive innervation of the mouse knee.[40] Na$_V$1.8, in particular, is highly localized to nociceptors[41] and, therefore, Na$_V$1.8-Cre can be used to label most of these neurons in mice. In young male mice (10 weeks old), innervation was observed in the lateral synovium, the connective tissue layer (the epiligament) surrounding the cruciate ligaments, and the insertion sites of the cruciate ligaments as well as dense innervation of bone marrow cavities. These neurons likely are mostly Aδ/C-type nociceptors, as reported previously in the literature.[41] Important changes in this pattern were observed 16 weeks after destabilization of the medial meniscus (DMM) surgery, a procedure that produces slowly developing OA-like joint damage and accompanying pain behaviors.[42] In association with joint damage in the medial compartment of the operated knee, fluorescently labeled nerves were noted in the synovium as well as increased innervation of the meniscus and major changes in the innervation of the subchondral bone. In particular, remodeling in the sclerotic subchondral bone was accompanied by densely innervated subchondral bone channels in the tibial plateaus and femoral condyles (for an example, see **Fig. 2**). Thus, these studies confirm immunohistochemical studies in human knees with end-stage knee OA and show that genetically labeled mice, such as these, can be used to document changes in joint innervation over time.

In recent years, Ca^{2+} imaging techniques of DRGs in live mice have been developed,[43] enabling visualization as a marker of electrical activity of L4-DRG neurons (where a majority of cell bodies of afferents coming from the knee and paw are located) in response to mechanical stimuli applied to the knee.[44] When the activity of knee-innervating DRG neurons is examined using this in vivo Ca^{2+} imaging technique, a noxious knee twist or knee pinch produces an increased number of activated neurons 8 weeks following DMM in comparison to sham surgery, indicating that this stimulus now recruits a population of newly sensitized neurons—possibly representing a category of previously silent nociceptors.[44–46] Increased responses to knee pinch have also been observed using this technique in the mouse anterior cruciate ligament transection model.[47] An important question is whether any of the plastic changes in knee innervation observed in OA, such as the neurons present in the subchondral bone channels or in the synovium and meniscus, correspond to these newly recruited

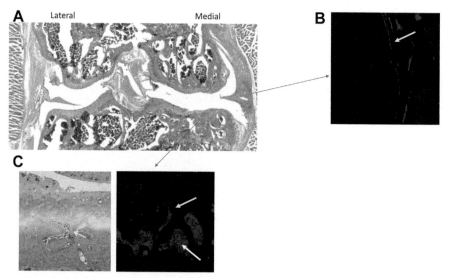

Fig. 2. (*A*) Using $Na_V1.8$ tdTomato reporter mice, hematoxylin-eosin staining (original magnification ×4) shows OA joint damage in the medial compartment 16 weeks after DMM; (*B*) new nociceptors are present in the medial synovium; (*C*) subchondral bone channels (*left* [*yellow arrow*]) contain $Na_V1.8$ nociceptors (*right* [*yellow arrow*]). The white arrow points to bone marrow cavities, which also are innervated. (*Data from* Obeidat AM, Miller RE, Miller RJ, Malfait AM: The nociceptive innervation of the normal and osteoarthritic mouse knee. Osteoarthritis Cartilage 2019, 27(11):1669-1679.)

previously silent nociceptors. If this is the case, they would provide a defined target for therapeutic intervention in OA pain, and their subtype could be molecularly defined, as discussed previously, in order to identify druggable targets expressed by these newly recruited neurons.

THE ROLE OF NERVE GROWTH FACTOR IN OSTEOARTHRITIS PAIN

An important development that has illuminated mechanisms underlying OA pain has been the discovery of the involvement of NGF signaling. The neurotrophin, NGF, was first identified as an important factor that regulates the growth and survival of both sympathetic and sensory neurons.[48] Mice where the *Ngf* gene is deleted show an extensive loss of sensory and sympathetic innervation and diminished response to noxious stimuli.[49] In humans, several mutations have been described in the *NGF* gene as well as in the gene encoding TrkA (*NTRK1*), and these mutations are associated with congenital insensitivity to pain, complicated by severe musculoskeletal manifestations, such as fractures and neuropathic joints (reviewed by Drissi and colleagues[3]). After development, NGF has been shown to have several important functions, both within and outside the nervous system; notably, it is a key protein for producing pain (reviewed by Denk and colleagues[50] and by Barker and colleagues[51]). NGF can exert its proalgesic actions through several different mechanisms. For example, it produces rapid excitatory effects in a subset of nociceptors that express its high-affinity receptor, TrkA. Activation of this receptor produces several rapid excitatory signaling events, such as transactivation, and increased expression of a variety of ion channels and receptors including the transient receptor vanilloid 1 (TRPV1), Na_Vs and calcium channels, acid-sensing ion channels, and mechanosensitive channels (discussed later).

Consistent with these effects, local injection of NGF produces immediate and often long-lasting pain responses in animals and humans (reviewed by Malfait and colleagues[52]). In healthy adults, for example, a single subcutaneous injection of recombinant NGF has been shown to elicit rapid-onset local injection-site hyperalgesia. This effect persists for up to 7 weeks.[53] Likewise, intradermal injection of NGF produces long-lasting local pressure allodynia.[54] The long-lasting effects suggest that they might be mediated by new nerve growth, and it was hypothesized that NGF-induced nerve growth might produce beneficial effects in certain neurodegenerative diseases, for example, in diabetic neuropathy, in which there is a marked degeneration of the cutaneous innervation.[55] The painful effects of NGF after injection in patients resulted, however, in cancellation of clinical trials that explored the use of NGF for this indication.[56] NGF produces pain on injection into the cervical facet joints of the spine.[57] When injected intra-articularly into the knee joints of healthy rats, it rapidly causes acute swelling and pain behaviors, including mechanical allodynia and weight-bearing deficits.[58,59] OA knees are more sensitive to the pain-inducing effects of NGF than healthy knees.[58]

Because of the clear ability of NGF to produce pain behaviors, it has been considered a good candidate as an essential algogenic mediator involved in several chronic painful diseases in humans. Consequently, neutralizing antibodies that sequester NGF and prevent it from binding to TrkA were developed, and clinical trials testing these antibodies have been going on for more than 20 years in conditions, such as chronic low back pain and OA (reviewed by Malfait and colleagues[52]). Of all these efforts, the beneficial effects of anti-NGF in OA have proved particularly marked. The anti-NGF antibody, tanezumab, is expected to be approved by the US Food and Drug Administration for the treatment of OA pain in the near future, in spite of the occurrence of rapidly progressive OA as a poorly understood side effect in a small percentage of people receiving the antibody (discussed by Malfait and colleagues[52]). Recently (October 1, 2020), anti-NGF antibodies were approved in Europe for alleviation of OA pain in dogs (https://www.ema.europa.eu/en/medicines/veterinary/summaries-opinion/librela). Blockade of NGF-TrkAs signaling also has shown analgesic effects in several rodent models of OA, with varying effects on joint health—although in-depth studies are lacking (reviewed by Malfait and colleagues[52] and by Vincent[60]). Irrespective of anything else, these observations clearly indicate that NGF signaling does play a role in enabling chronic OA pain. In addition, because these antibodies do not cross the blood-brain barrier, these findings further strongly support the idea that peripheral drive maintains pain in this disease. Consequently, elucidating exactly how NGF contributes to OA pain and how inhibiting its biological effects modifies pain pathways in OA—and also may affect joint integrity—will be of great importance for understanding the entire disease.

Clearly, NGF is present in joints affected by OA—for example, levels are higher in the synovial fluid in patients with knee OA than in controls,[61] and synovial fluid levels have been correlated with poor knee function.[62] Although it is known, however, that many cell types—including joint cells, such as chondrocytes, fibroblasts, and innate immune cells—can produce NGF in response to cytokine stimulation[63] (reviewed by Denk and colleagues[50]), it is not clear exactly which cells in osteoarthritic joints produce the neurotrophin. In surgical mouse models of OA, *Ngf* mRNA is up regulated in the whole joint,[64] specifically in articular cartilage[66] immediately after surgery and also in the late stage of the model, when mice show chronic pain. Recent work in human OA knee joints has reported NGF immunoreactivity in specific localizations associated with knee pain. Specifically, NGF immunoreactivity in the synovium, mostly in synovial fibroblasts and to a lesser extent in macrophages, was associated with pain.[66] Importantly, NGF expression in osteochondral channels as well as increased osteoclast density were associated with symptomatic knee OA, independently of synovitis or chondropathy.[67] NGF-like immunoreactivity in the subchondral bone was predominantly found associated with osteoclasts and mononuclear cells.[67]

There are several mechanisms through which anti-NGF antibodies could produce relief of OA pain. It is clear from studies using in vivo Ca^{2+} imaging to monitor the activity of $Na_V1.8$-expressing nociceptors that injection of NGF into the mouse knee produces immediate nociceptor excitation,[68] presumably due to its ability to depolarize these neurons through mechanisms, such as the transactivation of TRPV1 (discussed previously). In addition, NGF signaling modifies the properties of nociceptor ion channels, resulting in sensitization so that nerves are more likely to fire in response to normal mechanically driven stimuli associated with joint usage. Hence, ongoing release of NGF in OA can be expected to produce pain and inhibiting these actions to block these effects. During the past 2 decades, numerous ion channels, including acid-sensing ion channels, TRPA1, TRPC3, TRPC6, TACAN (also known as Tmem120 A), and PIEZO2, have been proposed to contribute to mechanosensitivity of sensory neurons. The biophysical properties of PIEZO2 appear well suited for mediating light touch (low threshold of activation and rapidly inactivating) and proprioception[69] rather than pain, whereas a channel with a high activation threshold that exhibits slow inactivation, such as TACAN, would seem more appropriate.[70] PIEZO2 has been shown expressed, however, by nociceptors and to play a role in mediating mechanical pain associated with models of inflammation and nerve injury[46,71–73]; so, how it may contribute to mechanical pain, particularly in disease states, is an area of active investigation. At this time, it is unclear which channels mediate mechanical depolarization of the nociceptor population involved in OA and how these may be related to the effects of NGF. An interesting set of observations demonstrated that application of NGF to DRG neurons in culture greatly increased their mechanosensitivity by sensitizing the activity of PIEZO2 mechanoreceptors in neurons.[46] These observations, therefore, might correspond to the increased activity of previously silent nociceptors observed in in vivo Ca^{2+} imaging studies, discussed previously. A precise description of the cellular populations of DRG neurons that express mechanosensitive channels, such as PIEZO2 and TACAN, as well as their colocalization with TrkA, clearly would be of interest, in order to increase understanding of the role NGF plays in the mechanical pain that is a feature of OA.

In addition to its acute actions that result in the functional sensitization of nociceptor populations, the continuous action of NGF in OA might well be responsible for the remodeling of the joint innervation observed in OA—although this has not yet been investigated directly. The authors recently found that injection of NGF into the mouse knee produces marked $Na_V1.8$ hyperinnervation of joint tissues, notably, the synovium and the subchondral bone (Obeidat and colleagues; unpublished data)—effects that are not surprising considering the well-known ability of NGF to support growth and survival of sensory neurons. The purpose of the anatomic remodeling of joint nociceptors in the OA joint, as described previously, is unclear. Anatomic remodeling may represent an attempt to produce neurogenic repair of the joint in the face of ongoing bone and cartilage degradation. At the same time, this enhanced nerve growth may provide a substrate for increased nociceptor activation and pain, which may be regarded as an injury-related signal for preventing joint usage and thus promote healing. If anti-NGF treatment also reduces enhanced nerve innervation of the joint, then this may well contribute to its antinociceptive actions, particularly with regard to the long-lasting nature of its effects in humans. It has been reported that administration of the small molecule TrkA inhibitor, AR786, reversed the appearance of CGRP-immunoreactive nerves in the osteochondral channels and reduced pain behaviors in rats with surgically induced OA,[39] an observation that further suggests the importance of these structures in OA pain.

It is not known at this point which of these NGF actions is most important for the observed analgesic effects of anti-NGF in OA, and it is conceivable that they both are involved during the progression of the disease. Furthermore, it also is possible that NGF sensitizes nociceptors indirectly through actions on non-neuronal cells in the joint. Not only do some populations of immune cells produce NGF—for example, in OA knee joints, NGF immunoreactive macrophages have been detected in the synovium, and this was correlated with pain[66]—but also others express TrkA and respond to NGF by releasing inflammatory cytokines, which then can further enhance nociceptor excitability by directly activating these neurons or through an action on other non-neuronal cells further elaborating an ever-expanding excitatory cytokine cascade. For example, in response to NGF, mast cells produce prostaglandin D2 that then can act on nociceptors, a mechanism which may contribute to mechanical allodynia in a mouse model of OA.[74] NGF also has been found to be present in, and released from, human $CD14^+$ T-cell clones and human monocytes. NGF has been shown to increase the release of mediators, including interleukin (IL)-1β, bradykinin, histamine, adenosine triphosphate, serotonin, and protons from inflammatory cells. Many non-neuronal cells, including bone and chondrocytes, also express mechanosensitive PIEZO channels whose activation may be linked to the synthesis and release of inflammatory cytokines.[75–77] Whether these PIEZO channels also can be sensitized by NGF as in sensory neurons (discussed previously) is not yet known, but this should be an important question to address in the context of a mechanically driven diseases, such as OA.

Study of the current literature, therefore, reveals that knowledge of the expression patterns and precise biological effects of NGF-TrkA signaling in the OA joint is limited. Importantly, the clinical trials with anti-NGF revealed that a small percentage of patients treated with the antibody developed rapidly progressive OA, which resulted in the need for joint replacement.[52,78] In view of this unexplained side effect, going forward it is important to paint an accurate picture of the entire NGF-TrkA interactome in the OA joint, detailing which cells express NGF and TrkA at which points in time during the development of the disease. Because the pain-relieving effects of anti-NGF are not in doubt, a detailed understanding of its mechanism of action certainly will help in understanding the basis of OA pain and also may provide insight into the relationship between pain and joint damage. Furthermore, the observed analgesic effects with targeting NGF-TrkA also may suggest novel strategies for targeting OA pain. If the precise identity of the neuronal subtypes involved in OA pain can be defined—and these may well be TrkA-expressing neurons (see **Fig. 1**)—then, because single-cell RNA sequencing can identify the receptome of these DRG neurons, targeting receptors that are particularly associated with these specific neurons may enable the selective inhibition of OA pain.

NEUROIMMUNE INVOLVEMENT IN OSTEOARTHRITIS PAIN

As described previously, the sensory nervous system is designed to perform its function of detecting potentially noxious stimuli and producing pain in order to help maintain homeostasis in the face of danger. One aspect of this response is that the nervous system is in constant communication not only with innervated tissues but also with the immune system—which also plays a vital role in the protection of organisms and the maintenance of homeostasis. The bidirectional cross-talk between the nervous system and the immune system currently is the focus of intense investigation as a major pathogenic contributor to the establishment and maintenance of chronic pain.[15,79] In cases of OA, emphasis is on the innate immune system, which increasingly is appreciated to play a role in driving joint damage and pain, as discussed in depth in several recent reviews.[17,80] One particular pathway that is shared by the innate immune and the sensory nervous system is mediated by pattern recognition receptors (PRRs) that can respond to signals provided by pathogens (pathogen-associated molecular patterns, such as microbial nucleic acids, lipoproteins, and carbohydrates) or damage-associated molecular patterns ([DAMPs], also known as alarmins, such as S100A8/9). These molecular patterns bind PRRs, such as toll-like receptors (TLRs), nucleotide oligomerization domain-like receptors, and the intracellular RNA-sensing retinoic acid–inducible gene I–like receptors, resulting in cellular responses that try to re-establish tissue homeostasis through triggering the synthesis of inflammatory cytokines and chemokines.[81] In the context of OA, it has been proposed that molecules arising from the degradation of joint tissues may activate TLRs expressed by nociceptors, resulting in direct excitation and pain. This has been shown for the TLR4 ligand, S100A8/9[82,83] as well as for a 32–amino acid aggrecan fragment that is released from cartilage when ADAMTS4/5 and matrix metalloproteinases degrade aggrecan in the interglobular domain.[84] This 32-mer aggrecan fragment can activate nociceptors through TLR2 and produce hyperalgesia following its injection into the knee cavity of naive mice. In vivo studies in mice have revealed that *Tlr4* null or *Tlr2* null mice develop joint damage after DMM surgery, but they are protected from knee hyperalgesia (Miller and colleagues[84] and unpublished data). These data, therefore, exemplify how a DAMP that is specific to OA cartilage damage can produce pain behavior through direct activation of DRG neurons. In contrast, *Tlr2* and *Tlr4* null mice are not protected from developing persistent mechanical allodynia, suggesting that many different pathways further contribute to the chronification of pain. Neuroimmune cross-talk at the level of the DRGs is thought to be key in maintenance of pain,[85] and, in the context of the DMM model, the authors recently reported a microarray study of the knee-innervating DRGs, where pathway analysis suggested a role for immune cell recruitment in this model.[86]

Neuroimmune pathways of pain generation can be amplified further when inflammatory cytokines synthesized as a result of TLR activation in resident and infiltrating joint cells, such as chondrocytes and macrophages, act on joint nociceptors directly—or on other joint tissues and immune cells, triggering further elements of an inflammatory cascade. It is clear that cytokines like IL-1, IL-6, IL-17, tumor necrosis factor α, and chemokines such as CCL2 can engage receptors expressed by nociceptors and trigger excitation and sensitization through variety of mechanisms, including TRP channel and Na_V transactivation.[87] In the cases of CCL2 and its receptor CCR2, a series of studies have demonstrated that these molecules are up-regulated following DMM and contribute to OA pain at defined points in the progression of the disease in this model.[88–90]

The possible role of DAMPs as mediators of OA pain clearly is an attractive possibility but needs further confirmation in both mice and humans. Furthermore, it is important to try t understand how such DAMP-mediated effects might be integrated into the developing narrative of NGF signaling in OA pain. This generally is true of all investigations directed at understanding the mechanisms of OA pain. Traditionally, the pharmacology of OA pain has been envisaged as developing particular targets, which can be modified by highly specific drugs and clearly this is part of the process. All of these targets, however, operate in the context of constantly shifting joint biology. Observations from human subjects and from animals using models, such as the DMM and monosodium iodoacetate models, clearly have indicated that the establishment of OA pain is a time-dependent process and that different biological processes, involving different molecular targets are operating during different phases of the disease (these temporal considerations were recently elegantly reviewed by Vincent[91]). Drugs that modify NGF-dependent joint innervation and drugs that modify neuroimmune or other influences may be appropriate at different stages of the disease in different patient populations. Future treatment of OA pain may constitute an array of targeted interventions designed to treat specific populations of patients. In order to develop these effective therapeutic approaches to OA pain, an accurate description of exactly how the disease develops from a cellular, molecular, and genetic perspective and how different populations of joint cells communicate with one another across space and time must continue to be established.

CLINICS CARE POINTS

- OA worldwide is one of the major causes of chronic pain. Currently available analgesic drugs fall short of patients' needs.
- Neutralizing antibodies targeting the neurotrophin, NGF, are in clinical development for OA pain. Trial results indicate that this is a highly promising biological therapy for OA pain, but a small proportion of patients treated with the antibodies develop rapidly progressive OA. The mechanism underlying this side effect is not understood.
- Neuroimmune interactions provide a rich substrate of potential targets for the development of new drugs for OA pain.

- Future treatment of OA pain may constitute an array of targeted interventions designed to treat specific populations of patients with OA.

ACKNOWLEDGMENTS

The authors thank the National Institutes of Health (National Institute of Arthritis and Musculoskeletal and Skin Diseases (NIAMS), grant numbers R01AR060364 to A.-M. Malfait and R01AR064251 to A.-M. Malfait, and R.J. Miller, and K01AR070328 to R.E. Miller. A.-M. Malfait is supported by the George W. Stuppy, MD, Chair of Arthritis at Rush University.

DISCLOSURE

AM Malfait has received consulting fees from Eli Lilly/Pfizer, as well as from Ceva and from Vizuri.

REFERENCES

1. Raja SN, Carr DB, Cohen M, et al. The revised International Association for the Study of Pain definition of pain: concepts, challenges, and compromises. Pain 2020;161(9):1976–82.
2. Woller SA, Eddinger KA, Corr M, et al. An overview of pathways encoding nociception. Clin Exp Rheumatol 2018;36(1):172.
3. Drissi I, Woods WA, Woods CG. Understanding the genetic basis of congenital insensitivity to pain. Br Med Bull 2020;133(1):65–78.
4. Emery EC, Luiz AP, Wood JN. Nav1.7 and other voltage-gated sodium channels as drug targets for pain relief. Expert Opin Ther Targets 2016;20(8):975–83.
5. Woolf CJ. Central sensitization: implications for the diagnosis and treatment of pain. Pain 2011;152(3 Suppl):S2–15.
6. Collaborators G. Global, regional, and national incidence, prevalence, and years lived with disability for 354 diseases and injuries for 195 countries and territories, 1990-2017: a systematic analysis for the Global Burden of Disease Study 2017. Lancet 2018;392(10159):1789–858.
7. Malfait AM, Schnitzer TJ. Towards a mechanism-based approach to pain management in osteoarthritis. Nat Rev Rheumatol 2013;9(11):654–64.
8. Arendt-Nielsen L. Pain sensitisation in osteoarthritis. Clin Exp Rheumatol 2017;35 Suppl 107(5):68–74.
9. Carlesso LC, Neogi T. Identifying pain susceptibility phenotypes in knee osteoarthritis. Clin Exp Rheumatol 2019;37 Suppl 120(5):96–9.
10. Roth BL. DREADDs for neuroscientists. Neuron 2016;89(4):683–94.
11. Miller RE, Ishihara S, Bhattacharyya B, et al. Chemogenetic inhibition of pain neurons in a mouse model of osteoarthritis. Arthritis Rheumatol 2017;69(7):1429–39.
12. Chakrabarti S, Pattison LA, Doleschall B, et al. Intraarticular adeno-associated virus serotype AAV-PHP.S-mediated chemogenetic targeting of knee-innervating dorsal root ganglion neurons alleviates inflammatory pain in mice. Arthritis Rheumatol 2020;72(10):1749–58.
13. Beswick AD, Wylde V, Gooberman-Hill R, et al. What proportion of patients report long-term pain after total hip or knee replacement for osteoarthritis? A systematic review of prospective studies in unselected patients. BMJ Open 2012;2(1):e000435.

14. Walsh DA. Editorial: arthritis pain: moving between early- and late-stage disease. Arthritis Rheumatol 2017;69(7):1343–5.
15. Hore Z, Denk F. Neuroimmune interactions in chronic pain - An interdisciplinary perspective. Brain Behav Immun 2019;79:56–62.
16. Chu C, Artis D, Chiu IM. Neuro-immune interactions in the tissues. Immunity 2020; 52(3):464–74.
17. Miller RJ, Malfait AM, Miller RE. The innate immune response as a mediator of osteoarthritis pain. Osteoarthritis Cartilage 2020;28(5):562–71.
18. Lluch E, Torres R, Nijs J, et al. Evidence for central sensitization in patients with osteoarthritis pain: a systematic literature review. Eur J Pain 2014;18(10): 1367–75.
19. Walsh DA, Stocks J. New therapeutic targets for osteoarthritis pain. SLAS Discov 2017;22(8):931–49.
20. Basbaum AI, Bautista DM, Scherrer G, et al. Cellular and molecular mechanisms of pain. Cell 2009;139(2):267–84.
21. Raja SN, Meyer RA, Campbell JN. Peripheral mechanisms of somatic pain. Anesthesiology 1988;68(4):571–90.
22. Woolf CJ, Ma Q. Nociceptors–noxious stimulus detectors. Neuron 2007;55(3): 353–64.
23. Emery EC, Ernfors P. Dorsal root ganglion neuron types and their functional specialization. Wood JN, editor. The oxford handbook of the neurobiology of pain. 2019. Oxford University Press, Oxford UK.
24. Lawson SN, Waddell PJ. Soma neurofilament immunoreactivity is related to cell size and fibre conduction velocity in rat primary sensory neurons. J Physiol 1991;435:41–63.
25. Averill S, McMahon SB, Clary DO, et al. Immunocytochemical localization of trkA receptors in chemically identified subgroups of adult rat sensory neurons. Eur J Neurosci 1995;7(7):1484–94.
26. McNeil B, Dong X. Mrgprs as itch receptors. In: Carstens E, Akiyama T, editors. Itch: mechanisms and treatment. Boca Raton (FL): CRC Press/Taylor & Francis; 2014.
27. Zylka MJ, Rice FL, Anderson DJ. Topographically distinct epidermal nociceptive circuits revealed by axonal tracers targeted to Mrgprd. Neuron 2005;45(1):17–25.
28. Liu Q, Tang Z, Surdenikova L, et al. Sensory neuron-specific GPCR Mrgprs are itch receptors mediating chloroquine-induced pruritus. Cell 2009;139(7): 1353–65.
29. Liu Q, Vrontou S, Rice FL, et al. Molecular genetic visualization of a rare subset of unmyelinated sensory neurons that may detect gentle touch. Nat Neurosci 2007; 10(8):946–8.
30. Usoskin D, Furlan A, Islam S, et al. Unbiased classification of sensory neuron types by large-scale single-cell RNA sequencing. Nat Neurosci 2015;18(1): 145–53.
31. Zeisel A, Hochgerner H, Lonnerberg P, et al. Molecular architecture of the mouse nervous system. Cell 2018;174(4):999–1014.e2.
32. Skoglund S. Anatomical and physiological studies of knee joint innervation in the cat. Acta Physiol Scand Suppl 1956;36(124):1–101.
33. Heppelmann B. Anatomy and histology of joint innervation. J Peripher Nerv Syst 1997;2(1):5–16.
34. McDougall JJ, Bray RC, Sharkey KA. Morphological and immunohistochemical examination of nerves in normal and injured collateral ligaments of rat, rabbit, and human knee joints. Anat Rec 1997;248(1):29–39.

35. Suri S, Gill SE, Massena de Camin S, et al. Neurovascular invasion at the osteo-chondral junction and in osteophytes in osteoarthritis. Ann Rheum Dis 2007; 66(11):1423–8.
36. Ashraf S, Wibberley H, Mapp PI, et al. Increased vascular penetration and nerve growth in the meniscus: a potential source of pain in osteoarthritis. Ann Rheum Dis 2011;70(3):523–9.
37. Mapp PI, Avery PS, McWilliams DF, et al. Angiogenesis in two animal models of osteoarthritis. Osteoarthritis Cartilage 2008;16(1):61–9.
38. Mapp PI, Sagar DR, Ashraf S, et al. Differences in structural and pain phenotypes in the sodium monoiodoacetate and meniscal transection models of osteoar-thritis. Osteoarthritis Cartilage 2013;21(9):1336–45.
39. Aso K, Shahtaheri SM, Hill R, et al. Contribution of nerves within osteochondral channels to osteoarthritis knee pain in humans and rats. Osteoarthritis Cartilage 2020;28(9):1245–54.
40. Obeidat AM, Miller RE, Miller RJ, et al. The nociceptive innervation of the normal and osteoarthritic mouse knee. Osteoarthritis Cartilage 2019;27(11):1669–79.
41. Shields SD, Ahn HS, Yang Y, et al. Nav1.8 expression is not restricted to nocicep-tors in mouse peripheral nervous system. Pain 2012;153(10):2017–30.
42. Miller RE, Malfait AM. Osteoarthritis pain: what are we learning from animal models? Best Pract Res Clin Rheumatol 2017;31(5):676–87.
43. Kim YS, Anderson M, Park K, et al. Coupled activation of primary sensory neu-rons contributes to chronic pain. Neuron 2016;91(5):1085–96.
44. Miller RE, Kim YS, Tran PB, et al. Visualization of peripheral neuron sensitization in a surgical mouse model of osteoarthritis by in vivo calcium imaging. Arthritis Rheumatol 2018;70(1):88–97.
45. Schmidt R, Schmelz M, Forster C, et al. Novel classes of responsive and unre-sponsive C nociceptors in human skin. J Neurosci 1995;15(1 Pt 1):333–41.
46. Prato V, Taberner FJ, Hockley JRF, et al. Functional and molecular characteriza-tion of mechanoinsensitive "silent" nociceptors. Cell Rep 2017;21(11):3102–15.
47. Zhu S, Zhu J, Zhen G, et al. Subchondral bone osteoclasts induce sensory inner-vation and osteoarthritis pain. J Clin Invest 2019;129(3):1076–93.
48. Cohen S, Levi-Montalcini R. Purification and properties of a nerve growth-promoting factor isolated from mouse sarcoma 180. Cancer Res 1957;17(1): 15–20.
49. Crowley C, Spencer SD, Nishimura MC, et al. Mice lacking nerve growth factor display perinatal loss of sensory and sympathetic neurons yet develop basal forebrain cholinergic neurons. Cell 1994;76(6):1001–11.
50. Denk F, Bennett DL, McMahon SB. Nerve growth factor and pain mechanisms. Annu Rev Neurosci 2017;40:307–25.
51. Barker PA, Mantyh P, Arendt-Nielsen L, et al. Nerve growth factor signaling and its contribution to pain. J Pain Res 2020;13:1223–41.
52. Malfait AM, Miller RE, Block JA. Targeting neurotrophic factors: novel approaches to musculoskeletal pain. Pharmacol Ther 2020;211:107553.
53. Petty BG, Cornblath DR, Adornato BT, et al. The effect of systemically adminis-tered recombinant human nerve growth factor in healthy human subjects. Ann Neurol 1994;36(2):244–6.
54. Dyck PJ, Peroutka S, Rask C, et al. Intradermal recombinant human nerve growth factor induces pressure allodynia and lowered heat-pain threshold in humans. Neurology 1997;48(2):501–5.

55. Hefti F, Hartikka J, Knusel B. Function of neurotrophic factors in the adult and aging brain and their possible use in the treatment of neurodegenerative diseases. Neurobiol Aging 1989;10(5):515–33.
56. Apfel SC. Nerve growth factor for the treatment of diabetic neuropathy: what went wrong, what went right, and what does the future hold? Int Rev Neurobiol 2002; 50:393–413.
57. Kras JV, Weisshaar CL, Pall PS, et al. Pain from intra-articular NGF or joint injury in the rat requires contributions from peptidergic joint afferents. Neurosci Lett 2015; 604:193–8.
58. Ashraf S, Mapp PI, Burston J, et al. Augmented pain behavioural responses to intra-articular injection of nerve growth factor in two animal models of osteoarthritis. Ann Rheum Dis 2014;73(9):1710–8.
59. Haywood AR, Hathway GJ, Chapman V. Differential contributions of peripheral and central mechanisms to pain in a rodent model of osteoarthritis. Sci Rep 2018;8(1):7122.
60. Vincent TL. Of mice and men: converging on a common molecular understanding of osteoarthritis. Lancet Rheumatol 2020;2(10):e633–45.
61. Montagnoli C, Tiribuzi R, Crispoltoni L, et al. beta-NGF and beta-NGF receptor upregulation in blood and synovial fluid in osteoarthritis. Biol Chem 2017; 398(9):1045–54.
62. Nees TA, Rosshirt N, Zhang JA, et al. Synovial cytokines significantly correlate with osteoarthritis-related knee pain and disability: inflammatory mediators of potential clinical relevance. J Clin Med 2019;8(9):1343.
63. Pecchi E, Priam S, Gosset M, et al. Induction of nerve growth factor expression and release by mechanical and inflammatory stimuli in chondrocytes: possible involvement in osteoarthritis pain. Arthritis Res Ther 2014;16(1):R16.
64. McNamee KE, Burleigh A, Gompels LL, et al. Treatment of murine osteoarthritis with TrkAd5 reveals a pivotal role for nerve growth factor in non-inflammatory joint pain. Pain 2010;149(2):386–92.
65. Driscoll C, Chanalaris A, Knights C, et al. Nociceptive sensitizers are regulated in damaged joint tissues, including articular cartilage, when osteoarthritic mice display pain behavior. Arthritis Rheumatol 2016;68(4):857–67.
66. Stoppiello LA, Mapp PI, Wilson D, et al. Structural associations of symptomatic knee osteoarthritis. Arthritis Rheumatol 2014;66(11):3018–27.
67. Aso K, Shahtaheri SM, Hill R, et al. Associations of symptomatic knee osteoarthritis with histopathologic features in subchondral bone. Arthritis Rheumatol 2019;71(6):916–24.
68. Ren D, Miller R, Malfait A, et al. Developing a functional imaging method for pharmacologically characterizing intra-articular sensory neurons. Orthopedic Research Society annual meeting (abstract) Feb 8-11. 2020:Phoenix AZ.
69. Murthy SE, Dubin AE, Patapoutian A. Piezos thrive under pressure: mechanically activated ion channels in health and disease. Nat Rev Mol Cell Biol 2017;18(12): 771–83.
70. Beaulieu-Laroche L, Christin M, Donoghue A, et al. TACAN is an ion channel involved in sensing mechanical pain. Cell 2020;180(5):956–67.e7.
71. Murthy SE, Loud MC, Daou I, et al. The mechanosensitive ion channel Piezo2 mediates sensitivity to mechanical pain in mice. Sci Transl Med 2018;10(462): eaat9897.
72. Szczot M, Liljencrantz J, Ghitani N, et al. PIEZO2 mediates injury-induced tactile pain in mice and humans. Sci Transl Med 2018;10(462):eaat9892.

73. Szczot M, Pogorzala LA, Solinski HJ, et al. Cell-type-specific splicing of Piezo2 regulates mechanotransduction. Cell Rep 2017;21(10):2760–71.

74. Sousa-Valente J, Calvo L, Vacca V, et al. Role of TrkA signalling and mast cells in the initiation of osteoarthritis pain in the monoiodoacetate model. Osteoarthritis Cartilage 2018;26(1):84–94.

75. Lee W, Leddy HA, Chen Y, et al. Synergy between Piezo1 and Piezo2 channels confers high-strain mechanosensitivity to articular cartilage. Proc Natl Acad Sci U S A 2014;111(47):E5114–22.

76. Servin-Vences MR, Moroni M, Lewin GR, et al. Direct measurement of TRPV4 and PIEZO1 activity reveals multiple mechanotransduction pathways in chondrocytes. Elife 2017;6:e21074.

77. Li X, Han L, Nookaew I, et al. Stimulation of Piezo1 by mechanical signals promotes bone anabolism. Elife 2019;8:e49631.

78. Hochberg MC, Tive LA, Abramson SB, et al. When is osteonecrosis not osteonecrosis?: Adjudication of reported serious adverse joint events in the tanezumab clinical development program. Arthritis Rheumatol 2016;68(2):382–91.

79. Jain A, Hakim S, Woolf CJ. Unraveling the plastic peripheral neuroimmune interactome. J Immunol 2020;204(2):257–63.

80. van den Bosch MHJ, van Lent P, van der Kraan PM. Identifying effector molecules, cells, and cytokines of innate immunity in OA. Osteoarthritis Cartilage 2020;28(5):532–43.

81. Newton K, Dixit VM. Signaling in innate immunity and inflammation. Cold Spring Harb Perspect Biol 2012;4(3):a006049.

82. Miller RE, Belmadani A, Ishihara S, et al. Damage-associated molecular patterns generated in osteoarthritis directly excite murine nociceptive neurons through Toll-like receptor 4. Arthritis Rheumatol 2015;67(11):2933–43.

83. Blom AB, van den Bosch MH, Blaney Davidson EN, et al. The alarmins S100A8 and S100A9 mediate acute pain in experimental synovitis. Arthritis Res Ther 2020;22(1):199.

84. Miller RE, Ishihara S, Tran PB, et al. An aggrecan fragment drives osteoarthritis pain through Toll-like receptor 2. JCI Insight 2018;3(6):e95704.

85. Raoof R, Willemen H, Eijkelkamp N. Divergent roles of immune cells and their mediators in pain. Rheumatology (Oxford) 2018;57(3):429–40.

86. Miller RE, Tran PB, Ishihara S, et al. Microarray analyses of the dorsal root ganglia support a role for innate neuro-immune pathways in persistent pain in experimental osteoarthritis. Osteoarthritis Cartilage 2020;28(5):581–92.

87. Miller RJ, Jung H, Bhangoo SK, et al. Cytokine and chemokine regulation of sensory neuron function. Handb Exp Pharmacol 2009;194:417–49.

88. Miller RE, Tran PB, Das R, et al. CCR2 chemokine receptor signaling mediates pain in experimental osteoarthritis. Proc Natl Acad Sci U S A 2012;109(50):20602–7.

89. Longobardi L, Temple JD, Tagliafierro L, et al. Role of the C-C chemokine receptor-2 in a murine model of injury-induced osteoarthritis. Osteoarthritis Cartilage 2017;25(6):914–25.

90. Miotla Zarebska J, Chanalaris A, Driscoll C, et al. CCL2 and CCR2 regulate pain-related behaviour and early gene expression in post-traumatic murine osteoarthritis but contribute little to chondropathy. Osteoarthritis Cartilage 2017;25(3):406–12.

91. Vincent TL. Peripheral pain mechanisms in osteoarthritis. Pain 2020;161:S138–46.

Targeting Nerve Growth Factor for Pain Management in Osteoarthritis—Clinical Efficacy and Safety

Brett W. Dietz, MD[a],*, Mary C. Nakamura, MD[b],
Matthew T. Bell, BS[c], Nancy E. Lane, MD[d]

KEYWORDS

- NGF • Anti-NGF • Osteoarthritis • Pain • Nerve growth factor • Review

KEY POINTS

- Nerve growth factor plays a key role in pain hypersensitization in osteoarthritis.
- Inhibition of nerve growth factor is effective at reducing pain and improving physical function from osteoarthritis of the hip or knee.
- Use of these agents is complicated by adverse joint safety events, notably rapidly progressive osteoarthritis and an increased need for joint replacements.
- The mechanism driving these joint safety events remains poorly understood and is an important area for further study.

BACKGROUND

Osteoarthritis (OA) is a leading cause of global disability,[1] affecting as many as 250 million people worldwide.[2] Estimates of the direct and indirect economic costs of OA range from 1% to 2.5% of the gross domestic product in the United States, Canada, France, the United Kingdom, and Australia.[3] Guidelines for management of OA generally agree on nonpharmacologic management with exercise, weight loss, education and self-management, and hip or knee joint replacement in appropriate patients. Pharmacologic agents that are variably recommended for management of OA include

[a] Division of Rheumatology, Department of Medicine, University of California, San Francisco, 400 Parnassus Avenue, Floor B1, San Francisco, CA 94143, USA; [b] Division of Rheumatology, Department of Medicine, University of California, San Francisco, San Francisco Veteran's Affairs Health Care System, 4150 Clement Street 111R, San Francisco, CA 94121, USA; [c] School of Medicine, St. Louis University, 1402 South Grand Boulevard, St Louis, MO 63104, USA; [d] Division of Rheumatology, Department of Internal Medicine, UC Davis Health, 4625 Second Avenue, Sacramento, CA 95917, USA
* Corresponding author.
E-mail address: brett.dietz@ucsf.edu

Rheum Dis Clin N Am 47 (2021) 181–195
https://doi.org/10.1016/j.rdc.2020.12.003
0889-857X/21/Published by Elsevier Inc.

acetaminophen, topical and oral nonsteroidal anti-inflammatory drugs (NSAIDs), duloxetine, tramadol, and intra-articular corticosteroids.[4] Due to concerns regarding limited and/or uncertain efficacy[5,6] and overall safety of many of these agents, their utility in OA management is limited. Nontramadol opioid medications have serious safety issues, may be less effective than nonopiates in OA, and generally are not recommended.[7] Given this significant unmet need for novel therapeutics, the development of additional effective nonopioid pain medications for OA and other conditions has been a topic of intense investigation, including compounds targeting nerve growth factor (NGF). The clinical efficacy and safety profile of these anti-NGF agents are the focus of this review.

BIOLOGIC ROLE OF NERVE GROWTH FACTOR

NGF is a member of a family of proteins called neurotrophins that regulate the development and survival of certain neurons. NGF is critical to the development of the peripheral sensory and sympathetic nervous system in mammals,[8,9] including humans.[10] NGF mediates its effects on the nervous system via signaling through 2 receptors: a specific tyrosine receptor kinase A (TrkA) (**Fig. 1**) and the low-affinity p75 neurotrophin receptor.[11] Humans with mutated NGF-B genes have congenital pain insensitivity,[10] and mutations in TrkA cause pain insensitivity, anhidrosis, and developmental delay.[12]

Aside from its profound developmental importance, NGF plays a role in pain signaling in adults. Injection of NGF induces hyperalgesic effects including heat sensitivity, myalgias and tenderness to palpation lasting weeks, and NGF expression has been associated with inflammatory, neuropathic, visceral, and cancer pain.[13] NGF is released by inflammatory cells in response to injury,[14] and appears to play an important role in pain and cachexia in pre-clinical models of inflammatory arthritis.[15] NGF also regulates levels of neuropeptides such as substance P and calcitonin gene-related peptide in adult sensory neurons.[16] NGF binding its TrkA receptor leads hypersensitization via several mechanisms, including rapid post-translational modifications

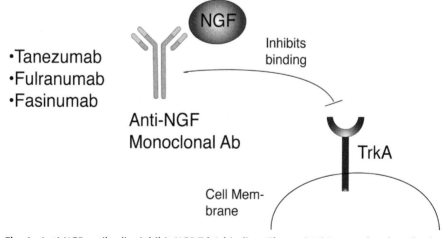

Fig. 1. Anti-NGF antibodies inhibit NGF-TrkA binding. The anti-NGF monoclonal antibodies tanezumab, fasinumab, and fulranumab bind to NGF and inhibit NGF interaction with its high-affinity receptor TrkA. The p75 receptor (not shown) is a low-affinity receptor that interacts with NGF. The p75 receptor can enhance NGF-TrkA interactions, although the precise interactions between TrkA and p75 are incompletely understood. Ab, antibody.

of ion channels, and increasing expression of a host of receptors in the membranes of sensory neurons.[17] A model of the effects of NGF on pain signaling is depicted in **Fig. 2**. NGF binds to TrkA, and the complex is endocytosed and retrogradely transported to neuronal cell bodies, where it modulates the expression of cell surface receptors involved in nociception in the dorsal root ganglion, thus initiating peripheral sensitization and pain hypersensitivity.[18,19]

NGF has effects beyond the nervous system. NGF-TrkA signaling in sensory nerves during late embryogenesis is required for normal vascularization and ossification of endochondral bone.[20] Sensory nerves emanating from the dorsal root ganglia extensively innervate the surfaces of mammalian bone. NGF/TrkA signaling in skeletal sensory nerves has been shown to be an early response to mechanical loading of bone. In vivo mechanical loading in mice and in vitro mechanical stretch were shown to induce profound up-regulation of NGF in osteoblasts. Elimination of TrkA signaling in mice was found to greatly attenuate load-induced bone formation whereas administration of exogenous NGF was found to significantly increase load-induced bone formation.[21]

Studies in mice and humans have suggested that there is a localized increase in NGF at sites of inflammation.[22] Human osteoarthritic chondrocytes in vitro demonstrate increased expression of TrkA and NGF-β protein relative to nonosteoarthritic chondrocytes, and the degree of expression increased with worsening osteoarthritic damage.[23] NGF is detectable in the synovial fluid of human patients with rheumatoid arthritis and OA but not in controls.[24] In different models of inflammation, NGF has

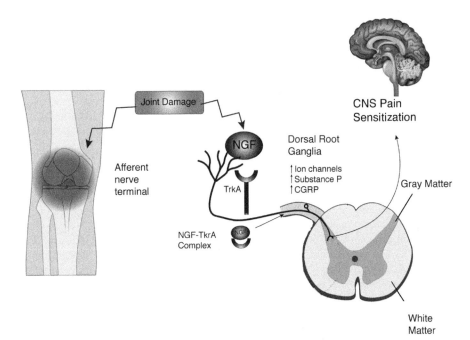

Fig. 2. NGF initiation of pain hypersensitization. NGF is released by damaged tissues and binds to its specific receptor, TrkA, on the terminals of sensory nociceptive neurons. The endocytosed NGF-TrkA complex is transported retrograde to the neuronal cell body in the dorsal root ganglion, where it increases expression of ion channels and neuropeptides, such as substance P and calcitonin gene–related peptide (CGRP), leading to peripheral and central pain hypersensitization. CNS, central nervous system.

been suggested to down-regulate tissue inflammation, including down-regulation of inflammatory cytokine production and up-regulation of the anti-inflammatory cytokine interleukin 10; thus, NGF may serve in part to dampen inflammatory responses to facilitate restoration of homeostasis.

NGF and its receptor, TrkA, appear also to regulate bone cells, including osteoblast[25] and osteoclast differentiation[26] and osteocyte activity[27] as well as homeostasis articular chondrocytes.[28] The role of neurotrophins on the differentiation and function of bone cells is an important area for further research, as better knowledge of this relationship and the interactions between bone cells, inflammatory cells, and sensory neurons is critical to understanding both the mechanism of action and the important adverse effects of anti-NGF agents.

NGF inhibitors in advanced phases of development for OA include tanezumab, a recombinant humanized anti-NGF monoclonal antibody,[29] and fasinumab, a recombinant fully human anti-NGF monoclonal antibody (**Table 1**).[30] Fulranumab, another human anti-NGF monoclonal antibody,[31] is discussed in later but is no longer in active development for OA.[32] These agents block the interaction of NGF with its receptors, TrkA and p75 (see **Fig. 1**).[29] Small-molecule selective TrkA inhibitors also are in development for OA pain[33] but have no published phase III data thus are not included in this review.

CLINICAL OUTCOMES IN ANTI–NERVE GROWTH FACTOR TRIALS

Many clinical trials of anti-NGF agents for hip and knee OA use scores on the Western Ontario and McMaster Universities Arthritis Index (WOMAC) as outcomes. The WOMAC is a self-administered patient-reported outcome instrument for OA of the hip or knee. It consists of 3 subscales (pain, stiffness, and physical function) covering 24 total items.[34] There are multiple versions of WOMAC and multiple scoring scales, including a 5-level Likert scale, 0 to 10 numeric rating scale (NRS), and 0 to 100 visual analog scale (VAS), leading to widely varying ranges of possible scores depending on the scale used and whether a total or average score is reported.[35] Least squares (LS) mean difference often is reported, which is the difference of group means after having adjusted for covariate(s). Whenever possible, the scale used in the referenced study are discussed.

EARLY-PHASE TRIALS OF ANTI–NERVE GROWTH FACTOR AGENTS FOR HIP OR KNEE OSTEOARTHRITIS

The initial studies of anti-NGF agents for OA of the hip or knee used intravenous (IV) formulations of tanezumab or fulranumab, each humanized anti-NGF antibodies, either alone or in combination with NSAIDs. In an early proof-of-concept study of tanezumab, 450 individuals with knee OA were randomized to receive IV tanezumab at various doses ranging from 10 μg/kg to 200 μg/kg for 2 administrations 8 weeks apart, compared with placebo. Averaged over 16 weeks, participants receiving tanezumab had reductions in WOMAC Pain score of 46% to 64% versus 23% for placebo, and reductions (indicating improvement) in the WOMAC Physical Function score of 47% to 65% versus 22% for placebo. Adverse events were common, especially at higher doses of tanezumab, 100 μg/kg and above, including headache, upper respiratory tract infection, and paresthesias.[36] A smaller phase II trial of 83 Japanese individuals with moderate to severe knee OA received a either single dose of IV tanezumab at doses ranging from 10 μg/kg to 200 μg/kg or placebo. At week 8, those receiving tanezumab, 25 μg/kg, 100 μg/kg, or 200 μg/kg, had improvement in WOMAC scores for pain (100-mm VAS; LS mean differences from placebo of −11.5, −9.6, −18.8,

Table 1
Summary of phase III trials of anti-nerve growth factor agents after lifting of Food and Drug Administration hold in 2015

Trial	Intervention	Follow-up	Results	Joint Adverse Events
Schnitzer et al,[55] 2019: TNZ for OA	698 patients randomized to TNZ, 2.5 mg, d 1; TNZ, 2.5 mg, wk 8; TNZ, 2.5 mg, d 1; TNZ, 5 mg, wk 8; or to PBO	40 wk	Both TNZ doses improved WOMAC Pain and Physical Function subscores and improved PGA-OA compared with PBO at 16 wk.	RPOA in 2.2% of TNZ, 2.5 mg/2.5 mg; 0.4% of TNZ, 2.5 mg/5 mg; 0% of PBO. TJR in 3.5% of TNZ, 2.5 mg/2.5 mg; 6.7% of TNZ, 2.5 mg/5 mg; 1.7% of PBO
Berenbaum et al,[56] 2020: TNZ for OA	849 patients randomized to TNZ, 2.5 mg; TNZ, 5 mg; or PBO, every 8 wk for 3 doses	48 wk	Both TNZ doses improved WOMAC Pain and Physical Function subscores compared with PBO at 24 wk. Only TNZ, 5 mg, was superior to PBO for PGA-OA at 24 wk.	RPOA in 1.4% of TNZ 2.5, mg; 2.8% of TNZ, 5 mg; 0% of PBO. TJR in 7.8% of TNZ, 2.5-mg; 7.0% TNZ, 5 mg; 6.7% PBO
Hochberg et al,[58] 2019: TNZ for OA	2996 patients randomized to TNZ, 2.5 mg, or TNZ, 5 mg, every 8 wk; or oral NSAID, up to wk 56	80 wk	TNZ, 5-mg dose, improved WOMAC Pain and WOMAC Physical Function at 16 wk compared with NSAIDs but no difference from NSAIDs at 56 wk. TNZ, 2.5 mg, not statistically different from NSAIDs at 16 wk or 56 wk	Composite joint safety outcome 3.8%, TNZ, 2.5 mg; 7.1%, TNZ 5 mg; 1.5% NSAIDs
Dakin et al,[59] 2019: FAS for OA	421 patients randomized to FAS, 1mg, 3mg, 6mg, or 9mg; or to PBO every 4 wk for 4 doses	36 wk	All FAS doses improved WOMAC Pain and Physical Function subscores compared with PBO at 16 wk. Only FAS, 1 mg and 9 mg, improved PGA-OA compared with PBO at 16 wk.	RPOA in 5% of fasinumab group (all doses averaged), 0% PBO. Subchondral insufficiency fracture in 1.8% fasinumab, 1.2% PBO. TJR 4% in both fasinumab and PBO
Markman et al,[62] 2020: TNZ for LBP	1832 patients randomized to TNZ, 5-mg SC; TNZ 10-mg SC; TRA; or PBO every 8 wk, up to wk 56	80 wk	TNZ, 10-mg dose, improved LBPI and RDQ score compared with PBO, and improved RDQ compared with TRA at 16 wk. TNZ, 5-mg dose, not statistically different from PBO at 16 wk	Composite adverse joint safety outcomes in 2.6% of TNZ, 10 mg; 1.0% of TNZ 5 mg; 0.2% of TRA

Abbreviations: FAS, fasinumab (subcutaneous); LBP, low back pain intensity; LBPI, low back pain intensity; NSAID, non-steroidal anti-inflammatory drug (oral); OA, osteoarthritis; PBO, placebo; TNZ, tanezumab (subcutaneous); TRA, tramadol (oral).

respectively) and physical function (100-mm VAS; LS mean differences from placebo of -8.7, -9.5, -17.6, respectively). Five study patients reported adverse events related to peripheral sensation, such as allodynia, paresthesia, thermohypoesthesia, and dysesthesia.[37] In summary, these phase II trials of tanezumab showed short-term efficacy in reducing pain and improving function in hip and knee OA, with adverse events of abnormal peripheral sensation.

Development of a different anti-NGF monoclonal antibody, fulranumab, occurred in parallel with the tanezumab trials. An early-phase study randomized 466 adults with moderate to severe OA pain of the hip or knee to receive subcutaneous fulranumab at various doses and frequencies, or placebo, both in addition to existing pain therapy. At week 12, those receiving the higher doses of fulranumab used in the study (3 mg every 4 weeks, 6 mg every 6 weeks, or 10 mg every 8 weeks) had improved WOMAC Pain subscale scores (0–10 NRS; LS mean differences from placebo -1.2, -0.8, and -0.9, respectively) and WOMAC Physical Function subscale scores (0–10 NRS; LS mean differences from placebo -1.3, -0.8, and -1.3, respectively). Neurologic adverse events were reported in 6% of the placebo group and 12% of patients treated with fulranumab, most commonly paresthesia and hypoesthesia.[31] In a phase II double-blind extension of the previous study, participants were eligible to continue to receive those doses of fulranumab throughout a 92-week extension phase, followed by a 24-week post-treatment follow-up period. The duration of drug exposure was less than planned due to a Food and Drug Administration (FDA) hold on the anti-NGF development program for joint-related adverse safety signals (discussed in more detail later). Efficacy data were summarized, however, up to week 49. By this point, the fulranumab, 3 mg every 4 weeks and 10 mg every 8 weeks, group had improvements in WOMAC Pain and Physical Function subscales versus placebo throughout the study. The safety analysis revealed a joint safety signal of rapidly progressive OA (RPOA) in 15 of the 388 people (3.8%) receiving fulranumab and in none of the placebo group. All cases of RPOA occurred in patients taking both fulranumab and NSAIDs.[38] Another trial of fulranumab as monotherapy compared with placebo or oxycodone was terminated early due to an FDA hold on the anti-NGF development program for adverse safety signals, but in the limited number of patients randomized, fulranumab-treated patients had better pain relief than with controlled-release oxycodone, but not better than placebo.[39] Taken together, the early studies of fulranumab showed efficacy at pain reduction with the higher doses, with adverse events similar to the tanezumab trials.

PRE–FOOD AND DRUG ADMINISTRATION HOLD PHASE III TRIALS OF ANTI–NERVE GROWTH FACTOR AGENTS FOR HIP OR KNEE OSTEOARTHRITIS

In the first phase III study of IV tanezumab for knee OA, 690 patients were randomized to receive a single dose of IV tanezumab at 2.5 mg, 5 mg, or 10 mg or placebo. In this and subsequent studies of tanezumab, the investigators used fixed-dose regimens rather than those based on body weight. At week 16, those receiving tanezumab, 2.5 mg, 5 mg, and 10 mg, had reductions in WOMAC Pain, WOMAC Physical Function, and patient global assessment (PGA) compared with placebo. Similar to prior studies, those receiving tanezumab had adverse events of abnormal peripheral sensation.[40] In the first phase III trial of tanezumab for hip OA, 627 participants were randomized to IV tanezumab at 2.5 mg, 5 mg, or 10 mg doses or placebo. At 16 weeks, each group receiving tanezumab had reduced WOMAC Pain, WOMAC Physical Function, and Patient Global Assessment of OA (PGA-OA) scores versus placebo. As with previous trials, the tanezumab groups had more adverse events compared with placebo, with abnormal peripheral sensation the most commonly reported.[41] This phase III placebo-controlled trial of IV tanezumab, therefore, showed efficacy at reducing OA pain and improving physical function, with a similar safety signal to the early-phase studies.

Additional phase III studies compared IV tanezumab to other analgesics. One phase III study randomized participants to tanezumab, 5 mg or 10 mg every 8 weeks for 1 or 2 doses; or controlled-release oxycodone; or placebo. At week 8, both the 5-mg and 10-mg tanezumab groups had improvement in the WOMAC Pain compared with placebo and oxycodone (0–10 NRS; LS mean differences from placebo −0.96 and −0.96, respectively, and LS mean differences from oxycodone −0.99 and −0.99, respectively, for tanezumab, 5 mg and 10 mg), improvement in the WOMAC Physical Function score (0–10 NRS; LS mean differences from placebo −1.14 and −1.15, respectively, and LS mean differences from oxycodone −1.00 and −1.01, respectively, for tanezumab, 5 mg and 10 mg), with similar rate of adverse peripheral sensation as in other studies and an overall lower rate of adverse events in tanezumab arms compared with oxycodone.[42] In 2 other randomized trials comparing IV tanezumab, 5 mg and 10 mg, against naproxen, 5-mg IV, tanezumab had superior improvement of WOMAC Pain score (0–10 NRS; LS mean differences −1.21 and −1.13 in 2 trials, respectively, vs placebo; LS mean differences −0.76 and −0.69 in 2 trials, respectively, vs naproxen), and improved WOMAC Physical Function and PGA over naproxen and placebo. The 10-mg IV tanezumab dose was only significantly better than naproxen for WOMAC Physical Function, not for WOMAC Pain or PGA. Overall rates of adverse events were similar for tanezumab and naproxen, although the 10-mg dose of tanezumab had more frequent peripheral abnormal sensation events.[11] These active-controlled phase III trials of IV tanezumab had short follow-up periods but demonstrated superior pain reduction and physical function with an overall favorable side-effect profile compared with opiate analgesics. When compared with oral NSAIDs, a typical first-line OA therapy, the results were mixed, with no superior pain relief at the higher tanezumab dose.

Additional studies examined the efficacy of IV tanezumab in combination with oral NSAIDs. In 1 study of individuals taking oral sustained-release diclofenac, 75 mg twice daily, for moderate to severe knee or hip OA, 607 participants were randomized to IV tanezumab, 2.5 mg, 5 mg, or 10 mg, or to placebo at weeks 0, 8, and 16. All continued diclofenac. At week 16, those receiving tanezumab and sustained-release diclofenac together had improvement over diclofenac plus placebo in WOMAC pain (0–10 NRS; LS mean differences from baseline −2.09, −2.19, and −2.25, respectively, and LS mean differences from placebo plus diclofenac −0.41, −0.51, and −0.57, respectively, in tanezumab, 2.5 mg, 5 mg, and 10 mg), with similar improvements in WOMAC Physical Function and PGA. The incidence of adverse events, however, was higher with combination therapy, including abnormal peripheral sensation, RPOA, and need for joint replacements.[43] Another study of patients with moderate to severe hip or knee OA expanded on these results by comparing tanezumab monotherapy with tanezumab combination therapy with NSAIDs versus NSAIDs treatment alone. In this study, 2700 individuals were randomized to receive IV tanezumab, 5 mg, 10 mg, or placebo, every 8 weeks, with or without oral naproxen or celecoxib. At 16 weeks, 5-mg and 10-mg tanezumab monotherapy improved WOMAC Pain and WOMAC Physical Function scores over NSAIDs alone, but no additional improvement was seen with combination therapy. Adverse events, however, were more frequent with tanezumab, especially with tanezumab and NSAIDs in combination, compared with NSAIDs therapy alone, primarily the development of RPOA.[44] Due to the high rate of adverse events seen in these combination trials of tanezumab and NSAIDs, and other trials of fulranumab in patients taking NSAIDs, in particular RPOA, the combination of anti-NGF agents and NSAIDs is not recommended.

SAFETY CONCERNS AND FOOD AND DRUG ADMINISTRATION HOLD

In 2010, after reports arose of adverse events classified as osteonecrosis in the phase II and phase III trials of tanezumab for low back pain and hip or knee OA, respectively, the FDA placed a partial clinical hold on tanezumab and, subsequently, all other anti-NGF monoclonal antibodies, including fulranumab, for all indications except for cancer pain. An adjudication committee was formed by Pfizer, the results of which were presented to the FDA in 2012. Janssen Research & Development conducted a similar process for fulranumab. In the 11,712 participants in the phase 3 OA and phase 2 chronic low back pain (cLBP) tanezumab development programs, there were 87 reported cases of osteonecrosis, 55 of which occurred when tanezumab and NSAIDs were used in combination, 28 in tanezumab monotherapy, 4 in active comparator agents, and 0 with placebo. After adjudication, most of the osteonecrosis adverse events were reclassified as worsening OA (58.6%), of which two-thirds were RPOA. In addition, 24.1% of the osteonecrosis events were reclassified as other diseases, the most common of which was a subchondral insufficiency fracture of the knee. Data from the phase II studies in the fulranumab development program revealed increased rate of total joint replacements in participants receiving fulranumab (86 per 1000 patient-years) than with oxycodone (39.8 per 1000 patient-years) or placebo (50.8 per 1000 patient-years). These reviews confirmed the adverse safety signal of RPOA and total joint replacements with use of anti-NGF monoclonal antibodies. The rate of these complications was greater with the higher doses of the anti-NGF antibodies and concurrent use of NSAIDs in combination with tanezumab. The vast majority (85%) of those receiving fulranumab already were receiving NSAIDs.[45,46]

After adjudication, most of the osteonecrosis events were reclassified as worsening or RPOA, and risk mitigation strategies were developed to reduce the risk of RPOA. These strategies included avoiding combination therapy with NSAIDs, using lower doses of anti-NGF agents administered subcutaneously, excluding patients with risk factors for RPOA or who would not be candidates for joint replacement, and establishing joint and neurologic safety monitoring protocols.[47] The FDA hold due to joint safety concerns was lifted in 2012.

Also in 2012, however, an additional clinical hold was placed due to reports of changes in the sympathetic nervous systems of animals receiving anti-NGF agents in nonclinical rodent studies. Three additional nonclinical studies of adult cynomolgus monkeys investigated the effect of subcutaneous tanezumab on the sympathetic nervous system. Tanezumab was associated with decreased sympathetic ganglia volume and average neuron size in the first month of treatment, but these changes were not associated with clinical deficits and reversed on drug withdrawal. There was no evidence found for adverse effects of sympathetic control of cardiovascular function (eg, orthostasis) nor evidence of neuronal cell death.[48] A study of fulranumab in adult cynomolgus monkeys similarly found decreased size of neurons and sympathetic ganglia, without evidence of neuronal cell death. The changes were found to be reversed after 3 months of drug withdrawal.[49] The clinical hold for sympathetic nervous system changes was lifted in 2015.

There is clinical evidence from case reports of skeletal disorders in some patients with congenital insensitivity to pain with anhidrosis, caused by loss-of-function mutations in either NGF or TrkA.[50–53] In these patients, fracture healing was described as occurring normally, but some patients developed a progressive arthropathy, resulting in disabling Charcot joints with gross deformity and instability. These patients lacked deep pain perception in bones and joints and had no protective reflexes, leading to significant bone and joint complications.[54]

POST-2015 PHASE III STUDIES IN KNEE AND HIP OSTEOARTHRITIS

Development of tanezumab and fasinumab resumed after lifting of the FDA holds in 2015. A summary of these post-2015 trials is provided in **Table 1**. In 1 phase III study, 698 participants with hip or knee OA who had not responded to or could not take standard OA analgesics were randomized to subcutaneous tanezumab, 2.5 mg, at week 1 and week 8; subcutaneous tanezumab, 2.5 mg, at week 1, and 5 mg at week 8; or placebo. At 16 weeks, WOMAC Pain scores (0–10 NRS) decreased from a mean of 7.1 to 3.6 in the tanezumab, 2.5-mg/2.5-m, group; from 7.3 to 3.6 in the tanezumab, 2.5-mg/5-m, group; and from 7.3 to 4.4 in the placebo arm (LS mean differences from placebo of −0.60 in the 2.5-mg/2.5-mg group and −0.73 in the 2.5-mg/5-mg group). There was a similar response in the WOMAC Physical Function score (0–10 NRS), with LS mean difference versus placebo of −0.66 for tanezumab, 2.5 mg/2.5 mg, and −0.89 for tanezumab, 2.5 mg/5 mg. Five patients in the tanezumab, 2.5-mg/2.5-m, arm (2.2%), and 1 patient in the tanezumab, 2.5-mg/5-m, arm (0.4%) developed RPOA versus no patients in the placebo group. Incidence rates of total joint replacement were 3.5%, 6.9%, and 1.7% in the tanezumab, 2.5-mg/2.5-mg; tanezumab, 2.5-mg/5-mg; and placebo groups, respectively.[55] In summary, lower doses of tanezumab administered subcutaneously reduced OA pain and improved function at 16 weeks but were associated with higher rates of RPOA and joint replacement compared to placebo.

Another phase III trial of subcutaneous tanezumab randomized 849 patients to receive tanezumab, 2.5 mg; tanezumab, 5 mg; or placebo every 8 weeks for 3 doses. At 24 weeks, the LS mean differences of tanezumab, 2.5 mg, compared with placebo was −0.46 for WOMAC Pain (0–10 NRS) and −0.59 for WOMAC Physical Function (0–10 NRS) but not significantly different than placebo for PGA-OA. For tanezumab, 5 mg, the LS mean differences from placebo were −0.62 for WOMAC Pain, −0.71 for WOMAC Physical Function, and −0.19 for PGA-OA (5-point Likert scale from 1 = very good to 5 = very poor). Safety findings were studied out to week 48. RPOA occurred in 0 patients receiving placebo; 4 patients (1.4%) receiving tanezumab, 2.5 mg; and 8 patients (2.8%) receiving tanezumab, 5 mg. There was 1 case of subchondral insufficiency fracture in the tanezumab, 2.5-mg group, and 1 case of primary osteonecrosis in the tanezumab, 5-mg, group. Rates of total joint replacement were 6.7% in placebo; 7.8% in tanezumab, 2.5 mg; and 7.0% in tanezumab, 5 mg. During the treatment period, paresthesia was more common with tanezumab, 5 mg (4.2%,) than with placebo (1.8%) and equivalent to placebo in tanezumab, 2.5 mg (1.8%). Hypoesthesia was more common in tanezumab, 5 mg (2.1%), and in tanezumab, 2.5 mg (1.4%), than in placebo (0.7%). None of the paresthesia or hypoesthesia events was considered severe. There were no patients in any of the groups who developed sympathetic neuropathies, as confirmed by protocol-specified cardiology or neurology consultation.[56] This study had a longer duration of treatment and monitoring than in previous studies and showed efficacy for pain and physical function of both 2.5-mg and 5-mg doses of subcutaneous tanezumab but with a dose-dependent increasing in adverse joint events compared with placebo.

Additional information on the long-term efficacy and safety of subcutaneous tanezumab for hip or knee OA comes from a phase III active-controlled study of subcutaneous tanezumab compared with NSAIDs, currently published in abstract form (NCT02528188). In this trial, 2996 participants who had moderate to severe hip or knee OA despite oral NSAIDs therapy either were switched to subcutaneous tanezu-mab or continued on oral NSAIDs. Patients received subcutaneous tanezumab (2.5 mg or 5 mg every 8 weeks) plus oral placebo, or oral NSAIDs plus subcutaneous placebo, continued from baseline through week 56, with an additional 24 weeks of safety monitoring. At week 16, those receiving tanezumab, 5 mg, had statistically significant improvement versus oral NSAIDs in WOMAC Pain (0–10 NRS; LS mean difference from NSAIDs −0.26) and in WOMAC Physical Function (0–10 NRS; LS mean difference from NSAIDs −0.31) but not in PGA-OA. The 2.5-mg tanezumab dose was not statistically different than NSAIDs therapy at week 16. Neither dose of tanezumab was statistically different than NSAIDs therapy at week 56.[57] The primary adjudicated composite joint safety outcome was defined as the combined rate of RPOA, osteonecrosis, subchondral insufficiency fracture, and pathologic fracture. At a total follow-up period of 80 weeks, the composite joint safety outcome occurred in 1.5% of the oral NSAIDs group; 3.8% of the tanezumab, 2.5-mg, group; and in 7.1% of the tanezumab, 5-mg, group. Most of these joint safety events were RPOA, occurring in 1.2% of the oral NSAIDs group; 3.2% of the tanezumab, 2.5-mg, group; and 6.3% in the tanezumab, 5-mg, group. Total joint replacement also was more common in tanezumab, 2.5 mg (5.3%), and in tanezumab, 5 mg (8.0%), than in those receiving oral NSAIDs (2.6%).[58] Although the lower dose of tanezumab, 2.5 mg, did not meet the efficacy endpoints versus oral NSAIDs in this study, the prolonged duration of treatment and follow-up provide the best information to date about the safety profile of tanezumab.

Fasinumab, a human anti-NGF monoclonal antibody, also is in phase III development. A phase IIb/III study randomized 421 individuals with hip or knee OA and inadequate response to analgesics to subcutaneous fasinumab at doses ranging from 1 mg to 9 mg every 4 weeks or placebo. At week 16, all doses of fasinumab led to decreased WOMAC Pain score (0–10 NRS; LS mean difference from placebo ranging from −0.8 to −1.4), with similar improvements in WOMAC Physical Function and PGA, with no obvious dose dependence observed. Adjudicated analysis found arthropathy adverse events in 5% of the study overall, involving 25 joints (13 index and 12 nonindex) in 7% of those in the fasinumab groups and 1% in the placebo group. The arthropathies demonstrated a dose relationship. RPOA occurred in 5% of the fasinumab and 0% of the placebo group, and subchondral insufficiency fractures in 1.8% of the fasinumab and 1.2% in the placebo group. The rates of joint replacement, approximately 4%, were similar in all groups. Most arthropathies were detected radiographically.[59]

As of the date of this publication, fulranumab is not in active development. Fasinumab is in ongoing phase III trials. The developer of tanezumab has submitted a biologics license application to the US Food and Drug Administration for the 2.5-mg dose of subcutaneous tanezumab for the treatment of moderate to severe OA.

ANTI–NERVE GROWTH FACTOR AGENTS FOR CHRONIC LOW BACK PAIN

Early studies of anti-NGF agents tanezumab, fulranumab, and fasinumab for cLBP showed mixed results in reducing pain versus placebo and shared the same joint safety concerns as in trials for hip and knee OA.[60] After lifting of the FDA hold in 2015, development of anti-NGF agents for cLBP resumed. Important outcome measures in these trials include the low back pain intensity (LBPI) score (0–10 NRS with 0 = no pain and 10 = most severe pain) and the Roland-Morris Disability Questionnaire (RDQ) (24-item assessment of daily physical function scored from 0 = no disability to 24 = maximum disability).[61]

The first phase III study of subcutaneous tanezumab randomized 1832 patients with cLBP and inadequate response to analgesics to receive subcutaneous tanezumab, 5 mg or 10 mg, every 8 weeks, or placebo, or prolonged-release oral tramadol. At 16 weeks, tanezumab, 10 mg, provided significantly better improvement in LBPI than placebo (LS mean difference vs placebo −0.40) and better improvement in RDQ than placebo (LS mean difference vs placebo −1.74). Improvements with tanezumab, 5 mg, were not significantly different than placebo at week 16. Neither tanezumab dose was superior to tramadol at reducing LBPI at 16 weeks, although tanezumab, 10 mg, provided greater reduction in RDQ than tramadol. There was no significant difference in LBPI or RDQ with tanezumab compared with placebo or tramadol at week 56. Joint safety adjudication revealed more frequent adverse joint safety outcomes in the tanezumab, 10-mg, group (2.6%) than in the tanezumab, 5-mg, group (1.0%), or than in the tramadol group (0.2%). The most frequent adverse joint outcome was RPOA (1.4% in the tanezumab, 10-mg, group) in 80 weeks' total follow-up.[62]

SUMMARY

NGF inhibitors reduce pain and improve physical function in patients with moderate to severe hip or knee OA. The anti-NGF antibodies currently under development are administered by subcutaneous injection every 4 weeks to 8 weeks, providing a prolonged duration of pain relief. Enthusiasm for these agents has been limited primarily by the development of RPOA and other adverse joint events that are dose-dependent safety signals seen with administration of anti-NGF agents, particularly because the mechanism behind these events is not entirely clear. The magnitude of and mechanism behind the further increased risk of RPOA when anti-NGF agents are combined with NSAIDs also are not defined. Relatively mild neurologic adverse events also have been reported. Trials have been relatively short term, and, given the chronic continuous nature of OA, the rates of RPOA and joint replacement during long-term use of anti-NGF agents also are not yet clear and remain areas of active investigation. In the largest recent studies, RPOA occurred in 2.4% to 8.4% of those receiving subcutaneous fasinumab at various doses for 16 weeks of treatment at 36 weeks' total follow-up[59]; in 3.2% of those receiving subcutaneous tanezumab, 2.5 mg; and 6.3% of those receiving tanezumab, 5 mg, for 56 weeks of treatment at 80 weeks' total follow-up.[58] Thus, the benefit of anti-NGF therapy to reduce pain and improve function must be balanced cautiously against the risk of accelerated OA. Further studies are needed to determine the mechanisms underlying the development of RPOA, which may enable identifying patients at higher or lower risk, which would enable a more personalized medicine approach to use of anti-NGF therapy.

CLINICS CARE POINTS

- Anti-NGF monoclonal antibodies are being considered for FDA approval for use in OA of the hip or knee.
- RPOA is a safety signal observed in NGF inhibitor trials that remains poorly understood.
- NGF inhibitors never should be used concurrently with NSAIDs due to an enhanced risk of RPOA when both agents are used together.
- The benefit of anti-NGF therapy to reduce pain and improve function must be balanced cautiously against the risk of accelerated OA.

DISCLOSURE

Dr B. Dietz and Dr M.C. Nakamura are supported by the Department of Veterans Affairs. Dr M.C. Nakamura is supported by the Department of Veterans Affairs Biomedical Laboratory R&D Merit Award BX002994, National Institute on Aging and Musculoskeletal and Skin Diseases Awards R01AR066735 and P30AR070155, and the Russell/Engelman Rheumatology Research Center at UCSF. Dr N.E. Lane has consulted for Pfizer and was a clinical investigator for the phase II and phase III studies with tanezumab.

REFERENCES

1. Cross M, Smith E, Hoy D, et al. The global burden of hip and knee osteoarthritis: estimates from the global burden of disease 2010 study. Ann Rheum Dis 2014; 73(7):1323-30.
2. Hunter DJ, Bierma-Zeinstra S. Osteoarthritis. Lancet 2019;393(10182):1745-59.
3. March LM, Bachmeier CJ. Economics of osteoarthritis: a global perspective. Baillieres Clin Rheumatol 1997;11(4):817-34.
4. Nelson AE, Allen KD, Golightly YM, et al. A systematic review of recommendations and guidelines for the management of osteoarthritis: the chronic osteoarthritis management initiative of the U.S. bone and joint initiative. Semin Arthritis Rheum 2014;43(6):701-12.
5. da Costa BR, Reichenbach S, Keller N, et al. Effectiveness of non-steroidal anti-inflammatory drugs for the treatment of pain in knee and hip osteoarthritis: a network meta-analysis. Lancet 2017;390(10090):e21-33.
6. Jüni P, Hari R, Rutjes AWS, et al. Intra-articular corticosteroid for knee osteoarthritis. Cochrane Database Syst Rev 2015;10:CD005328.
7. Deveza LA, Hunter DJ, Van Spil WE. Too much opioid, too much harm. Osteoarthritis Cartilage 2018;26(3):293-5.
8. Ritter AM, Lewin GR, Kremer NE, et al. Requirement for nerve growth factor in the development of myelinated nociceptors in vivo. Nature 1991;350(6318):500-2.
9. Crowley C, Spencer SD, Nishimura MC, et al. Mice lacking nerve growth factor display perinatal loss of sensory and sympathetic neurons yet develop basal forebrain cholinergic neurons. Cell 1994;76(6):1001-11.
10. Einarsdottir E, Carlsson A, Minde J, et al. A mutation in the nerve growth factor beta gene (NGFB) causes loss of pain perception. Hum Mol Genet 2004;13(8): 799-805.
11. Chao MV. Neurotrophins and their receptors: a convergence point for many signalling pathways. Nat Rev Neurosci 2003;4(4):299-309.
12. Indo Y. Molecular basis of congenital insensitivity to pain with anhidrosis (CIPA): mutations and polymorphisms in TRKA (NTRK1) gene encoding the receptor tyrosine kinase for nerve growth factor. Hum Mutat 2001;18(6):462-71.
13. Mizumura K, Murase S. Role of nerve growth factor in pain. In: Schaible H-G, editor. Pain Control. Handbook of experimental pharmacology. Berling, Heidelberg: Springer; 2015. p. 57-77. https://doi.org/10.1007/978-3-662-46450-2_4.
14. Lindholm D, Heumann R, Meyer M, et al. Interleukin-1 regulates synthesis of nerve growth factor in non-neuronal cells of rat sciatic nerve. Nature 1987; 330(6149):658-9.
15. Shelton DL, Zeller J, Ho W-H, et al. Nerve growth factor mediates hyperalgesia and cachexia in auto-immune arthritis. Pain 2005;116(1-2):8-16.
16. Lindsay RM, Harmar AJ. Nerve growth factor regulates expression of neuropeptide genes in adult sensory neurons. Nature 1989;337(6205):362-4.

17. Mantyh PW, Koltzenburg M, Mendell LM, et al. Antagonism of Nerve Growth Factor-TrkA Signaling and the Relief of Pain. Anesthesiology 2011;115(1): 189–204.
18. McKelvey L, Shorten GD, O'Keeffe GW. Nerve growth factor-mediated regulation of pain signalling and proposed new intervention strategies in clinical pain management. J Neurochem 2013;124(3):276–89.
19. Shang X, Wang Z, Tao H. Mechanism and therapeutic effectiveness of nerve growth factor in osteoarthritis pain. Ther Clin Risk Manag 2017;13:951–6.
20. Tomlinson RE, Li Z, Zhang Q, et al. NGF-TrkA signaling by sensory nerves coordinates the vascularization and ossification of developing endochondral bone. Cell Rep 2016;16(10):2723–35.
21. Tomlinson RE, Li Z, Li Z, et al. NGF-TrkA signaling in sensory nerves is required for skeletal adaptation to mechanical loads in mice. Proc Natl Acad Sci U S A 2017;114(18):E3632–41.
22. Minnone G, De Benedetti F, Bracci-Laudiero L. NGF and its receptors in the regulation of inflammatory response. Int J Mol Sci 2017;18(5). https://doi.org/10.3390/ijms18051028.
23. Iannone F, De Bari C, Dell'Accio F, et al. Increased expression of nerve growth factor (NGF) and high affinity NGF receptor (p140 TrkA) in human osteoarthritic chondrocytes. Rheumatology (Oxford) 2002;41(12):1413–8.
24. Aloe L, Tuveri MA, Carcassi U, et al. Nerve growth factor in the synovial fluid of patients with chronic arthritis. Arthritis Rheum 1992;35(3):351–5.
25. Johnstone MR, Brady RD, Schuijers JA, et al. The selective TrkA agonist, gambogic amide, promotes osteoblastic differentiation and improves fracture healing in mice. J Musculoskelet Neuronal Interact 2019;19(1):94–103.
26. Hemingway F, Taylor R, Knowles HJ, et al. RANKL-independent human osteoclast formation with APRIL, BAFF, NGF, IGF I and IGF II. Bone 2011;48(4):938–44.
27. Stapledon CJM, Tsangari H, Solomon LB, et al. Human osteocyte expression of nerve growth factor: the effect of pentosan polysulphate sodium (PPS) and implications for pain associated with knee osteoarthritis. PLoS One 2019;14(9): e0222602.
28. Jiang Y, Tuan RS. Role of NGF-TrkA signaling in calcification of articular chondrocytes. FASEB J 2019;33(9):10231–9.
29. Abdiche YN, Malashock DS, Pons J. Probing the binding mechanism and affinity of tanezumab, a recombinant humanized anti-NGF monoclonal antibody, using a repertoire of biosensors. Protein Sci 2008;17(8):1326–35.
30. Tiseo PJ, Kivitz AJ, Ervin JE, et al. Fasinumab (REGN475), an antibody against nerve growth factor for the treatment of pain: results from a double-blind, placebo-controlled exploratory study in osteoarthritis of the knee. Pain 2014; 155(7):1245–52.
31. Sanga P, Katz N, Polverejan E, et al. Efficacy, safety, and tolerability of fulranumab, an anti-nerve growth factor antibody, in the treatment of patients with moderate to severe osteoarthritis pain. Pain 2013;154(10):1910–9.
32. Janssen announces discontinuation of fulranumab phase 3 development program in osteoarthritis pain | Johnson & Johnson. Available at: https://www.jnj.com/media-center/press-releases/janssen-announces-discontinuation-of-fulranumab-phase-3-development-program-in-osteoarthritis-pain. Accessed October 21, 2020.
33. Walsh DA, Neogi T. A tale of two TrkA inhibitor trials: same target, divergent results. Osteoarthritis Cartilage 2019;27(11):1575–7.
34. Bellamy N, Buchanan WW, Goldsmith CH, et al. Validation study of WOMAC: a health status instrument for measuring clinically important patient relevant

outcomes to antirheumatic drug therapy in patients with osteoarthritis of the hip or knee. J Rheumatol 1988;15(12):1833–40.

35. Copsey B, Thompson JY, Vadher K, et al. Problems persist in reporting of methods and results for the WOMAC measure in hip and knee osteoarthritis trials. Qual Life Res 2019;28(2):335.

36. Lane NE, Schnitzer TJ, Birbara CA, et al. Tanezumab for the treatment of pain from osteoarthritis of the knee. N Engl J Med 2010;363(16):1521.

37. Nagashima H, Suzuki M, Araki S, et al. Preliminary assessment of the safety and efficacy of tanezumab in Japanese patients with moderate to severe osteoarthritis of the knee: a randomized, double-blind, dose-escalation, placebo-controlled study. Osteoarthritis Cartilage 2011;19(12):1405–12.

38. Sanga P, Katz N, Polverejan E, et al. Long-term safety and efficacy of fulranumab in patients with moderate-to-severe osteoarthritis pain: a phase ii randomized, double-blind, placebo-controlled extension study. Arthritis Rheumatol 2017; 69(4):763–73.

39. Mayorga AJ, Wang S, Kelly KM, et al. Efficacy and safety of fulranumab as monotherapy in patients with moderate to severe, chronic knee pain of primary osteoarthritis: a randomised, placebo- and active-controlled trial. Int J Clin Pract 2016; 70(6):493–505.

40. Brown MT, Murphy FT, Radin DM, et al. Tanezumab reduces osteoarthritic knee pain: results of a randomized, double-blind, placebo-controlled phase III trial. J Pain 2012;13(8):790–8.

41. Brown MT, Murphy FT, Radin DM, et al. Tanezumab reduces osteoarthritic hip pain: results of a randomized, double-blind, placebo-controlled phase III trial. Arthritis Rheum 2013;65(7):1795–803.

42. Spierings ELH, Fidelholtz J, Wolfram G, et al. A phase III placebo- and oxycodone-controlled study of tanezumab in adults with osteoarthritis pain of the hip or knee. Pain 2013;154(9):1603–12.

43. Balanescu AR, Feist E, Wolfram G, et al. Efficacy and safety of tanezumab added on to diclofenac sustained release in patients with knee or hip osteoarthritis: a double-blind, placebo-controlled, parallel-group, multicentre phase III randomised clinical trial. Ann Rheum Dis 2014;73(9):1665–72.

44. Schnitzer TJ, Ekman EF, Spierings ELH, et al. Efficacy and safety of tanezumab monotherapy or combined with non-steroidal anti-inflammatory drugs in the treatment of knee or hip osteoarthritis pain. Ann Rheum Dis 2015;74(6):1202–11.

45. Hochberg MC. Serious joint-related adverse events in randomized controlled trials of anti-nerve growth factor monoclonal antibodies. Osteoarthritis Cartilage 2015;23:S18–21.

46. Hochberg MC, Tive LA, Abramson SB, et al. When is osteonecrosis not osteonecrosis?: adjudication of reported serious adverse joint events in the tanezumab clinical development program. Arthritis Rheumatol Hoboken NJ 2016;68(2): 382–91.

47. Bélanger P, West CR, Brown MT. Development of pain therapies targeting nerve growth factor signal transduction and the strategies used to resolve safety issues. J Toxicol Sci 2018;43(1):1–10.

48. Belanger P, Butler P, Butt M, et al. From the cover: evaluation of the effects of tanezumab, a monoclonal antibody against nerve growth factor, on the sympathetic nervous system in adult cynomolgus monkeys (Macaca fascicularis): a stereologic, histomorphologic, and cardiofunctional assessment. Toxicol Sci 2017; 158(2):319–33.

49. Rocca M, Han C, Butt M, et al. Evaluation of the toxicity and neurological effects of fulranumab in adult cynomolgus monkeys. Int J Toxicol 2019. https://doi.org/10.1177/1091581819830980.

50. Rosemberg S, Marie SK, Kliemann S. Congenital insensitivity to pain with anhidrosis (hereditary sensory and autonomic neuropathy type IV). Pediatr Neurol 1994;11(1):50–6.

51. Toscano E, della Casa R, Mardy S, et al. Multisystem involvement in congenital insensitivity to pain with anhidrosis (CIPA), a nerve growth factor receptor(Trk A)-related disorder. Neuropediatrics 2000;31(1):39–41.

52. Indo Y, Mardy S, Miura Y, et al. Congenital insensitivity to pain with anhidrosis (CIPA): novel mutations of the TRKA (NTRK1) gene, a putative uniparental disomy, and a linkage of the mutant TRKA and PKLR genes in a family with CIPA and pyruvate kinase deficiency. Hum Mutat 2001;18(4):308–18.

53. Bonkowsky JL, Johnson J, Carey JC, et al. An infant with primary tooth loss and palmar hyperkeratosis: a novel mutation in the NTRK1 gene causing congenital insensitivity to pain with anhidrosis. Pediatrics 2003;112(3 Pt 1):e237–41.

54. Minde J, Svensson O, Holmberg M, et al. Orthopedic aspects of familial insensitivity to pain due to a novel nerve growth factor beta mutation. Acta Orthop 2006;77(2):198–202.

55. Schnitzer TJ, Easton R, Pang S, et al. Effect of tanezumab on joint pain, physical function, and patient global assessment of osteoarthritis among patients with osteoarthritis of the hip or knee. JAMA 2019;322(1):37–48.

56. Berenbaum F, Blanco FJ, Guermazi A, et al. Subcutaneous tanezumab for osteoarthritis of the hip or knee: efficacy and safety results from a 24-week randomised phase III study with a 24-week follow-up period. Ann Rheum Dis 2020;79(6):800–10.

57. Subcutaneous tanezumab vs NSAID for the treatment of osteoarthritis: efficacy and general safety results from a randomized, double-blind, active-controlled, 80-week, phase-3 study. ACR meeting abstracts. Available at: https://acrabstracts.org/abstract/subcutaneous-tanezumab-vs-nsaid-for-the-treatment-of-osteoarthritis-efficacy-and-general-safety-results-from-a-randomized-double-blind-active-controlled-80-week-phase-3-study/. Accessed October 20, 2020.

58. Subcutaneous tanezumab versus NSAID for the treatment of osteoarthritis: joint safety events in a randomized, double-blind, active-controlled, 80-week, phase-3 study. ACR meeting abstracts. Available at: https://acrabstracts.org/abstract/subcutaneous-tanezumab-versus-nsaid-for-the-treatment-of-osteoarthritis-joint-safety-events-in-a-randomized-double-blind-active-controlled-80-week-phase-3-study/. Accessed October 20, 2020.

59. Dakin P, DiMartino SJ, Gao H, et al. The efficacy, tolerability, and joint safety of fasinumab in osteoarthritis pain: a phase IIb/III double-blind, placebo-controlled, randomized clinical trial. Arthritis Rheumatol Hoboken NJ 2019;71(11):1824–34.

60. Leite VF, Buehler AM, El Abd O, et al. Anti-nerve growth factor in the treatment of low back pain and radiculopathy: a systematic review and a meta-analysis. Pain Physician 2014;17(1):E45–60.

61. Roland M, Morris R. A study of the natural history of back pain. Part I: development of a reliable and sensitive measure of disability in low-back pain. Spine 1983;8(2):141–4.

62. Markman JD, Bolash RB, McAlindon TE, et al. Tanezumab for chronic low back pain: a randomized, double-blind, placebo- and active-controlled, phase 3 study of efficacy and safety. Pain 2020;161(9):2068–78.

Pain in Axial Spondyloarthritis
Insights from Immunology and Brain Imaging

Ejaz M.I. Pathan, MD, PhD, MRCP[a],*,
Robert D. Inman, MD, FRCPC, FRCP Edin[b,c,d,e]

KEYWORDS

- Spondyloarthritis • Pain • Dynamic pain connectome • Neuro-immune interface

KEY POINTS

- Immune cells interact with neurons to modulate pain through either peripheral or central sensitization depending on the site of this interaction.
- The default mode network, salience network, and antinociceptive system exhibit functional connectivity, which modulates pain perception in this condition.
- Differences in pain perception in males and females have been demonstrated both in animal models as well as on neuroimaging.

INTRODUCTION

Back pain, which is worse at rest but better with exercise, of more than 3 months in duration, in individuals younger than 45 years, is typical of spondyloarthritis (SpA).[1] Other characteristic features include alternating buttock pain or pain that awakens in the second half of the night.[2] In clinical practice though, it is not uncommon for patients to present with pain that does not always fit this description, making it difficult to establish a diagnosis early in these patients. The increased use of MRI in the diagnosis of SpA has helped identify these patients earlier but also led to an understanding that these patients may also suffer with coexisting degenerative disk disease and that both of these factors could contribute to pain.[3] The Bath Ankylosing Spondylitis Index (BASDAI), which is meant to measure disease activity in SpA, does not distinguish between inflammatory and mechanical back pain.[4,5] Imaging has also highlighted the fact that patients who experience symptoms with SpA do not always show evidence

[a] Rheumatology Department, Freeman Hospital, Newcastle upon Tyne Hospitals NHS Foundation Trust, Freeman Road, High Heaton, Newcastle upon Tyne NE7 7DN, UK; [b] Spondylitis Program, Toronto Western Hospital, University Health Network, 399 Bathurst Street, Toronto, Ontario M5T 2S8, Canada; [c] Schroeder Arthritis Institute, University Health Network; [d] Department of Medicine, University of Toronto, Toronto, Ontario, Canada; [e] Department of Immunology, University of Toronto, Toronto, Ontario, Canada
* Corresponding author.
E-mail address: e.pathan@nhs.net

Rheum Dis Clin N Am 47 (2021) 197–213
https://doi.org/10.1016/j.rdc.2020.12.007

of active inflammatory lesions on MRI, as suggested by a recent study that showed no significant differences in Spondyloarthritis Research Consortium of Canada MRI scores in patients with low or high clinical disease activity scores.[6] Patients treated with biologic agents may show a response to treatment with lesions improving on MRI but do not disappear.[7] Pain in SpA is hence complex, multifactorial, and poorly understood.

There are also sex differences in SpA with women more likely to present with higher levels of pain.[8] Some argue that the presence of coexisting fibromyalgia may play a role in response to therapy.[9] Other factors, such as depression and anxiety, as well as sleep disorders, are common in SpA[10] and may also impact the individual's response to therapy. Functional MRI studies have recently shown the complex network of areas in the brain that are responsible for perception of pain in SpA.[11] An understanding of the differences in the immune response between the sexes has also helped better understand the difference in perception of pain and response to therapy.[12]

In this review, we describe recent advances in neuroimaging of various brain networks involved in pain in SpA. We also discuss the interface between the immune system and nervous system and how this leads to differences in pain perception between the sexes.

SOURCES OF PAIN IN AXIAL SPONDYLOARTHRITIS

Typically, the onset of pain in axial SpA is usually in the low back and is caused by inflammation of the sacroiliac joints. This may be due to synovitis, osteitis, or enthesitis at the sacroiliac joints.[13] Patients complain of alternating buttock pain, which is often responsive to nonsteroidal anti-inflammatory drugs (NSAIDs). Inflammation in the spine, seen as osteitis leading to hyperintense corner lesions at vertebral corners may be responsible for pain in other parts of the spine. Apart from osteitis, enthesitis, particularly of the anterior longitudinal ligament in the spine, and spondylodiscitis may be the cause of spinal pain.[14] In addition to the spine, inflammation of the costovertebral joints may cause anterior chest wall pain with reduced chest expansion and pain on deep inspiration.

A study comparing imaging to the site of pain, established a good correlation between site of pain and sacroiliitis but not between site of pain and spinal lesions on MRI.[15]

Later in the disease, development of syndesmophytes, as well as bony bridges, may be sources of pain. Despite excessive bone deposition, these patients are at risk of osteoporosis resulting in vertebral fractures with acute-onset back pain. Degenerative spine disease such as disk disease and spinal canal stenosis, as well as facet joint arthritis may be as common in this group of patients as it is in the general population and can coexist with inflammatory changes in the same patient.[16] Rarely, neurologic complications, such as atlanto-axial dislocation[17] or cauda equina syndrome,[18] may be seen in advanced cases. Apart from the structural causes listed previously, there have been some recent reports of cold hyposensitivity, mediated by Aδ fibers and reduced proprioception, mediated by Aβ fibers, in SpA suggesting the presence of neuropathic pain in SpA.[19]

Emotional factors, such as anxiety and depression, also may play a role in pain modulation in these patients.[10] Patients with comorbid fibromyalgia often exhibit higher pain scores and report higher overall scores on their Bath indices.[20] Patients with SpA with comorbid fibromyalgia are less likely to continue their first biologic.[21] They also tend to report only a modest response to therapy in terms of patient-reported outcomes although still show a similar drop in C-reactive protein levels.

Fatigue, poor work productivity, and poor quality of life are commonly associated with comorbid fibromyalgia.[9]

PAIN PERCEPTION

Nociceptors (somatosensory neurons that are sensitive to noxious stimuli) innervate the skin, muscles, joints, and periosteum carrying impulses via either fast-conducting Aδ myelinated fibers or slow-conducting nonmyelinated C fibers.[22] Although most nociceptors are polymodal, some are modality-specific, such as C-heat nociceptors and C-mechano-cold nociceptors.[23] Joints also show mechano-receptors that may not be sensitive to mechanical stimuli in the absence of tissue injury. However, when joints become inflamed, these silent receptors become active and mechanosensitive, and are also called mechanically insensitive afferents.[24] These mechanoreceptors have low thresholds similar to non-nociceptor mechanoreceptors, but in the presence of inflammation, there is a reduction in the action potential leading to pain sensitivity and hyperalgesia.[25]

L-glutamate is the primary neurotransmitter of nociceptors. Nociceptors are generally of 2 types, depending on the neurotransmitter released at synapse-peptidergic or non-peptidergic.[26] Neuropeptides such as either Substance P or Calcitonin gene-related peptide (CGRP) and expression of nerve growth factor (NGF) receptor tyrosine kinase A is found in peptidergic neurons. They also show presence of transient receptor potential vanilloid 1 (TRPV1) and transient receptor potential ankyrin 1 (TRPA1) channels. Non-peptidergic nociceptors express c-Ret, the receptor for glial cell line–derived neurotrophic factors, IB4 isolectin, and express purinergic P2X3 receptor.[26] Peptidergic nociceptors serve both afferent and efferent function and are hence known as sensorimotor nerves. They release Substance P and CGRP at the site of tissue injury leading to vasodilation, increased vascular permeability, and release of mediators from mast cells, also known as neurogenic inflammation.[27]

Although cartilage does not show any evidence of nerve fibers, an abundance of neuropeptide, Substance P, has been reported in periosteum, subchondral bone, bone marrow, fat pad, and joint capsule in patients with knee osteoarthritis.[28] Bone marrow edema has been shown to be a predictor of pain in temporomandibular osteoarthritis,[29] knee osteoarthritis, osteonecrosis, reflex sympathetic dystrophy, bone contusion after trauma, and stress fractures.[30] Similar bone edema is reported in both axial[31] and peripheral SpA.[32] Low threshold mechanoreceptors, mechanically sensitive nociceptors, and silent nociceptors have been shown in facet joints on neurophysiological studies.[33] Immunohistochemistry studies of cadaveric sacroiliac joints have also demonstrated the presence of neurotransmitters Substance P and CGRP.[34] Similarly, high levels of glutamate and its N-methyl D-Aspartate (NMDA) receptor, as well as Substance P, were found on immunohistochemistry in patients with patellar tendinopathy when compared with patients with tibial shaft fractures as controls.[35]

PAIN TRANSMISSION

Noxious stimuli lead to depolarization of the nociceptor leading to activation of Transient Receptor Potential channel subtypes (TRPA, TRPM, and TRPV), Sodium channel isoforms (Nav), Potassium channel subtypes (KCNK), and acid-sensing ion channels, releasing either glutamate or neuropeptides such as Substance P or CGRP and conduction of action potentials along type A and C fibers. These then communicate with second-order neurons in the dorsal horn of the spinal cord. Second-order neurons in turn decussate in the spinal cord and join the ascending fibers of the anterolateral system projecting to the brainstem and thalamus. Third-order neurons from the thalamus project to a number of different cortical and sub-cortical areas including the somatosensory cortex encoding sensory discriminative functions; anterior cingulate cortex, amygdala, and insular cortex encoding emotional responses; as well as prefrontal cortex encoding cognitive aspects of pain. Descending pathways modulating pain involve brainstem areas such as the peri-aqueductal gray, locus ceruleus, and rostral ventro-medial medulla.[36]

THE NEUROIMMUNE INTERFACE

Pain is a protective mechanism against tissue injury. The presence of inflammation leads to injury and is associated with pain. Resolution of inflammation in turn leads to resolution of pain, suggesting a link between the immune and nervous systems. Cytokines, lipids, proteases, and growth factors released from immune cells bind to receptors on nociceptors.[25] This binding causes activation of ion channels on the nociceptors and generation of pain impulses. In mouse models, cytokines and Prostaglandin E2 (PGE2) are released by neutrophils that migrate to the site of injury.[37] Activated mast cells that are associated with nociceptors in the mucosa on electron microscopy, release interleukin (IL)-5, IL-6, tumor necrosis factor (TNF)α, IL-1β as well as histamine, 5HT and NGF.[38] Cytokines, growth factors, and lipids are also released from macrophages and monocytes migrating to the injury site.[39,40] IL-17 A and interferon (IFN)γ released by T cells bind their receptors on nerve endings inducing pain.[41] Apart from nerve endings, immune cells also interact with the body of the nociceptors within the dorsal root ganglion with increased numbers of these cells in the dorsal root ganglion (DRG) after chemotherapy[42] and after sciatic nerve ligation induced pain[41] in animal models.

Cytokines may also activate nociceptors directly (**Table 1**).[25] p38 Membrane Associated Protein Kinase (MAPK) phosphorylation of Nav 1.8 sodium channels by IL-1β, leads to thermal hyperalgesia.[43] It can also lead to increased TRPV1 expression by activation of IL-1R on nociceptors and hence increases pain sensitivity to thermal stimuli. IL-6 binds gp-130 leading to increased expression of both TRPV1 and TRPA1.[44,45] Prostaglandins induced as a result, activate Prostaglandin EP1-EP4 receptors leading to sensitization of nociceptors to pain. Similarly, TNFα causes increased expression of TRPV1 and TRPA1 by p38 MAPK phosphorylation of Nav 1.8 and Nav 1.9 sodium channels leading to neuronal production of prostaglandins and hyperalgesia.[46–48] IL-6 induces mechanical hyperalgesia and IL-1β induces thermal hyperalgesia but TNFα induces both mechanical and thermal hyperalgesia.[49] A fast increase in neuronal excitability has been shown to be induced by IL-17A. This hypernociceptive effect has been shown to be blocked in antigen-induced arthritis mouse models by either pharmacologic or genetic inhibition of TNFα, IL-1β, CXCL1, endothelin-1, and prostaglandins.[50]

Nociceptors express chemokine receptors such as CC chemokine receptor 1 (CCR1) and CXC chemokine receptor 5 (CXCR5).[51] They also express receptors for prostaglandins and leukotrienes as well as for histamine. NGF, produced by immune cells during inflammation, can increase nerve density of the inflamed area and increase sensitivity to pain. It also produces increased oxidized lipid TRPV1 agonists and TRPV1 activity leading to persistent nociception.[52]

Nociceptors also exhibit pattern recognition receptors (PRRs) that recognize pathogen-associated molecular patterns and damage-associated molecular patterns. These PRRs include Toll-Like Receptors (TLRs) 2, 4, and 5 expressed on the cell surface, and TLRs 3, 7, and 9 expressed on endosomes, lysosomes, and the

Table 1
Sensitization of nociceptors by cytokines secreted by immune cells

Immune Cell	Cytokine Released	Receptor on Nerve Terminal	Channel Activated
Mast cells	IL-5	IL-5R	
	5-HT	5-HT2	
	Histamine	H1/2	
	NGF	TrkA	Nav1.7 & TRPV1
Mast cells, neutrophils, and macrophages	TNF α	TNF R1	Nav 1.8 & 1.9
	IL-1β	IL-1R	TRPV1
	LTB4	BLT1	
	IL-6	gp130	TRPV1 &TRPA1
Neutrophils and macrophages	PGE2	EP1-4	
Th 17 T cells	IL-17A	IL-17AR	

Immune cells, their mediators, and corresponding receptors on neurons responsible for peripheral sensitization. Inflammation leads to macrophages, monocytes, neutrophils, mast cells, as well as T cells accumulating at sites of inflammation. These cells release various mediators, including cytokines, growth factors, and prostaglandins, which in turn act on their respective receptors on neurons activating sodium channel isoforms (Nav) as well as Transient Receptor Potential cation channel subfamily vanilloid member 1 (TRPV1) and Transient Receptor Potential cation channel subfamily ankyrin member 1 (TRPA1). This leads to the depolarization of the neurons and increased sensitivity to noxious stimuli leading to hyperalgesia. Tumor necrosis factor (TNFα) binds to TNF α receptor 1 (TNFR1); interleukin (IL)-1b, which binds to IL-1 receptor (IL-1R); IL-6, which binds to gp130; prostaglandin (PG)E2, which binds to its receptor EP1-4; and leukotriene B4, which binds its receptor BLT1. In addition, mast cells secrete IL-5, which binds to IL-5 receptor (IL-5R); 5-HT, which binds to 5HT2 receptor; histamine and nerve growth factor (NGF), which bind to histamine receptor 2 (HR2) and tyrosine kinase A (TrkA) on the neuron, respectively. A subset of T cells, Th17 cells, also secrete IL-17A, which binds to IL-17A receptor (IL-17AR).

endoplasmic reticulum.[53] Cells within the nervous system such as microglia, astrocytes, oligodendrocytes, Schwann cells, satellite glial cells, fibroblasts, endothelial cells, macrophages, and sensory neurons have been shown to express TLRs. Cytokines and other soluble mediators that act on glial cells and neurons, induced by binding of TLR to its ligand, produces nociceptive hypersensitivity. ATP, which is detected by P2 purinergeic receptors, is a potent danger signal released following cell injury. Inotropic (P2X) receptors are ligand gated while metabotropic (P2Y) receptors are G-Protein coupled.[54] P2X receptors in neurons and microglia become permeable to ions leading to their activation. Sensitization of TRP and voltage-gated sodium channels in P2Y receptors contributes to nociceptor activation.

CENTRAL SENSITIZATION

Apart from nociceptors, potentiation of neurons in supraspinal areas like brainstem, thalamus, and cortex also leads to chronic pain. Activation of the immune system leads to disruption of the balance between excitatory and inhibitory processes.[55] Although this type of sensitization can be seen with nerve injury and inflammation, it also occurs in dysfunctional pain such as in fibromyalgia. These chronic pain states are associated with expansion of the receptive field such that there is an increased response to stimuli even on remote noninflamed normal tissues.[56]

Microglia have been shown to play a role in nociception.[57] Colony Stimulating Factor 1 (CSF1) released from afferent nerve fibers binds CSF1 receptor on microglia[58] inducing upregulation of ATP-sensitive P2X4 receptors on microglia in the spine.[59]

This in turn leads to activation of p38 MAP Kinase and secretion of signaling molecule Brain Derived Neurotrophic Factor (BDNF) at the synapse.[60] BDNF binds to tropomyosin receptor kinase (TRBK) on neurons in the dorsal horn of the spinal cord. This leads to downregulation of potassium-chloride cotransporter 2 (KCC2) and the phosphorylation of N-methyl-D-aspartate receptor (NMDAR) on neurons in the spinal cord transmitting signals to the brain.[61] This is required for the potentiation of NMDAR signaling. The resultant decreased inhibition and enhanced neuronal excitability results in neuropathic pain (**Fig. 1**A). The preceding process of expression of BDNF that results in sensitization of postsynaptic neurons by microglial cells has been shown in male mice. The same process is mediated by T cells infiltrating the spinal cord in female mice.[62]

Another mechanism of central sensitization is via TLR4-mediated release of inflammatory cytokines from microglia and astrocytes after chemotherapeutic cisplatin,[63] intraplantar formalin,[64] or intrathecal lipopolysaccharide (LPS) administration in mice models.[65] Activated TLR4 localizes to lipid rafts, the integrity of which is essential for TLR4 dimerization before initiation of the signaling cascade.[66–68] Removal of cholesterol from lipid rafts by Apolipoprotein A-I binding protein (AIBP) hence inhibits TLR4 signaling, which in turn reverses or prevents allodynia induced in mouse models.[69] Spinal delivery of AIBP in mouse models has been shown to significantly reduce levels of IL-6, IL-8, CCL2, and CXCL2 induced by intrathecal LPS as well as glial fibrillary acidic protein (GFAP) and ionized calcium binding adaptor molecule 1 (IBA1), markers of astrocyte and microglial activation suggesting that AIBP inhibits microglial activation in the spinal cord and may have therapeutic potential (**Fig. 1**B).[69]

Other glial cells, such as astrocytes and oligodendrocytes, also secrete inflammatory mediators like CX3CL1. This activates production of TNFα in a MAPK-dependent manner, leading to activation of spinal cord astrocytes. This in turn produces CCL2 in a JNK MAPK-dependent mechanism. CCL2 activates central neurons through CCR2 resulting in neuropathic pain.[70] Spinal cord oligodendrocytes produce IL-33, which activates microglia and astrocytes in mice hence contributing to chronic pain.[71]

SEXUAL DIFFERENCES IN CHRONIC PAIN

Mouse models show differences between male and female mice when subjected to intrathecal LPS.[72] LPS activates TLR4 in the spinal cord to induce mechanical allodynia only in male mice, but when LPS was administered in the brain or the hind paw, there was no difference between the sexes. Given that TLR4 is expressed on microglial cells, a further study showed that the microglial cells were only involved in inducing mechanical allodynia in male mice, while in female mice, adaptive immune cells such as T cells mediated the same function.[62] TAK 242, a TLR4 antagonist, was found in vitro to be effective in blocking the release of TNF from macrophages of both male and female C57Bl/6 mice treated with intrathecal LPS.[64] In the same study, intrathecal LPS-induced tactile allodynia to a greater extent in male mice, and deficiency of TLR4 as well as treatment with TAK242 reduced the allodynia more in males than females. The effect of TAK242 on preventing delayed tactile allodynia, studied by injecting intraplantar formalin, however, was the same in both males and females.

Another molecule that binds TLR4 is Spinal high mobility group box 1 protein (HMGB1), a non-histone nuclear protein, that plays an important role in both inflammation and pain processing.[73] It is reported to have a pronociceptive role in the spinal cord, DRG, and local peripheral tissues in experimental pain models of rheumatoid

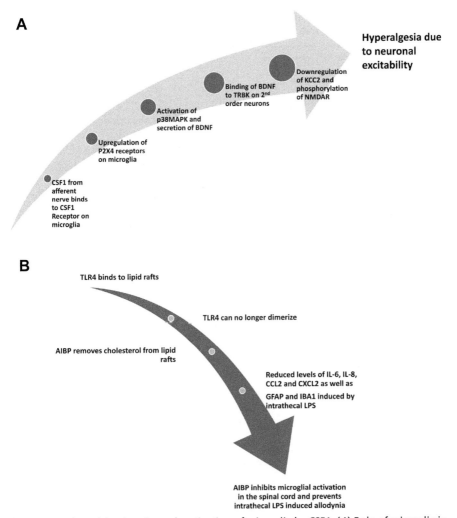

Fig. 1. Central sensitization through activation of microglia by CSF1. (*A*) Role of microglia in central sensitization of second-order neurons leading to hyperalgesia. In animal models, nerve injury results in the release of CSF1 from afferent nerve fibers, which binds CSF1 receptor on microglia. This in turn induces upregulation of ATP-sensitive P2X4 receptors on microglia in the spine leading to the activation of p38 MAP kinase and secretion of the signaling molecule BDNF, at the synapse. BDNF binds to tropomyosin receptor kinase (TRK) on neurons in the dorsal horn of the spinal cord causing downregulation of KCC2 and the phosphorylation of NMDAR on neurons in the spinal cord, thereby transmitting signals to the brain. Downregulation of KCC2 is required for the potentiation of NMDAR signaling. The resulting decreased inhibition and enhanced neuronal excitability result in neuropathic pain. The preceding process of expression of BDNF, which results in sensitization of postsynaptic neurons, has been shown to be mediated by T cells infiltrating the spinal cord in female mice, in contrast to the same process being mediated by microglial cells in male mice. Inhibition of central sensitization by AIBP through reduced microglial activation. (*B*) Another mechanism of central sensitization is via TLR4-mediated release of inflammatory cytokines from microglia and astrocytes after chemotherapeutic cisplatin, intra-plantar formalin or intrathecal LPS administration in mice models. Activated TLR4 localizes to lipid rafts, the integrity of which is essential for TLR4 dimerization prior to initiation of the

arthritis (RA).[74] The disulfide form of HMGB1, formed during inflammation, acts on TLR4 and induces cytokine production in both male and female mice.[75] However, the disulfide form of HMGB1 when injected into ankles, showed a delayed, yet longer lasting increase in mRNA of TNFα, IL1-β, IL-6, and CCL2 without inducing cellular infiltration in the ankle joints, suggesting it worked on tissue resident cells.[76] Inhibition of resident macrophages by Minocycline, reduced HMGB1-induced pain-like behavior only in male mice. Although TLR4 on nociceptors are important for HMGB1-induced pain in both sexes, the contribution of TLR4 on myeloid cells to nociception was minimal in females compared with males.[76]

In humans, 2 double-blind placebo-controlled studies from the same center showed LPS-induced systemic inflammation increases pain sensitivity was more pronounced in women as compared with men.[77] Although it is postulated that this may be sex-hormone related, no conclusive evidence of this association has been found. A study from our center of patients with ankylosing spondylitis (AS) showed sexual dimorphism with increased activation of Th17 axis in males but not females.[12] Further work is needed to understand if this difference plays a part response to therapy with IL-17 blockers.

From a clinical perspective, women show lower pain thresholds and greater temporal summation to brief repetitive stimuli than men.[78] However, they show greater adaptation to sustained noxious suprathreshold stimuli or habituation to longer sustained stimuli. Further work is needed to better understand the difference in pain perception between the sexes. Some insight into differences have become apparent from brain imaging. as discussed in the next section.

BRAIN IMAGING IN CHRONIC PAIN

Over the past decade, advances in structural and functional brain imaging have led to a better understanding of chronic pain. Depending on whether scanning involves a task, functional MRI (fMRI) scans are either stimulus or task evoked or resting state (task free).

An increase in blood flow related to increased neural activity can be detected on fMRI as Blood Oxygen Level Dependent signal, a measure of difference in magnetic properties between oxygenated and deoxygenated hemoglobin.[79] Although resting state or task-free fMRIs identify ultra-low frequency functional connectivity between brain regions, stimulus-evoked fMRI scans demonstrate how the brain reacts to noxious or non-noxious stimuli in chronic pain states. Another fMRI technique uses arterial spin labeling to monitor regional cerebral blood flow, which helps understand brain activity in a focal area related to ongoing spontaneous pain as seen in most chronic pain states.[80]

Structural MRI scans use techniques such as Voxel-based morphometry and cortical thickness analysis to quantify gray matter. Diffusion tensor imaging or tractography is another useful MRI technique to study white matter connectivity, using the difference in magnetic properties of tissues in which diffusion of water is either restricted

---

signaling cascade. Removal of cholesterol from lipid rafts by AIBP, hence inhibits TLR4 signaling, which in turn reverses or prevents allodynia induced in mouse models. Spinal delivery of AIBP in mouse models has been shown to significantly reduce levels of IL-6, IL-8, CCL2 and CXCL2 induced by intrathecal LPS as well as GFAP and IBA1, markers of astrocyte and microglial activation suggesting that AIBP inhibits microglial activation in the spinal cord and may have therapeutic potential.

or unrestricted. This measures fractional anisotropy on a scale between 0 and 1, where 0 represents unrestricted diffusion and 1 represents complete anisotropic diffusion.[80]

In chronic pain, the brainstem, insula, the primary and secondary somatosensory cortex, anterior and mid-cingulate cortex as well as the prefrontal cortex show altered stimulus-evoked and task-evoked responses on fMRI.[80] Abnormalities are also noted in the response and connectivity of the default mode network, salience network, and sensorimotor network. The anterior insula, medial cingulate cortex, temporoparietal junction, and dorsolateral prefrontal cortex together form the salience network. This network is more strongly activated by a noxious stimulus when the subject is paying attention to the painful stimulus. The posterior cingulate cortex, medial prefrontal cortex, lateral parietal, and area in the medial temporal lobe together form the default mode network (DMN). This network is active at rest or when attention is diverted but is suppressed when the subject is paying attention to painful stimulus. On the other hand, the antinociceptive system or the descending pain modulatory system that connects the medial prefrontal cortex of DMN and periaqueductal gray in the brainstem, shows more connectivity when the subject's attention is diverted. Individual differences in perception to pain may be accounted for by this system with those exhibiting low intrinsic attention to pain showing higher connectivity between the DMN and periaqueductal gray and others exhibiting high intrinsic attention to pain showing poorer connectivity. The dynamic nature of connectivity between the various brain regions altered with chronic pain had led to the coining of the term dynamic pain connectome (**Fig. 2**).[81]

Structural changes such as thinning of the medial cingulate cortex and anterior insula in irritable bowel syndrome[82] or thalamic gray matter volume changes in

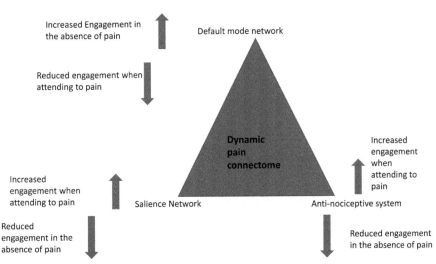

Fig. 2. Brain networks involved in pain perception. In the absence of pain, the DMN is found to be more engaged, observed on imaging. However, when exposed to a noxious stimulus, the SN and antinociceptive network show increased engagement, whereas the DMN shows reduced engagement. When attention is diverted away from pain, increased engagement of the DMN is again seen with increased functional connectivity between the prefrontal cortex of the DMN and the periaqueductal gray of the antinociceptive system.

temporomandibular joint dysfunction have also been reported.[83] These changes correlate to the duration of pain in these patients. Similar reversal of changes has also been shown in patients with chronic low back pain,[84] as well as patients undergoing hip replacement for osteoarthritis of the hips where pain resolved postoperatively.[85]

Hemodynamic-based fMRI has a temporal resolution of seconds and hence does not pick up faster occurring brain activity.[86] However, electroencephalography (EEG) or magnetoencephalography (MEG) detects abnormalities in the temporal resolution of milliseconds. These techniques show slower resting peak alpha frequency (PAF) in healthy individuals indicates greater pain sensitivity during pain.[87] Intensity of ongoing chronic pain has been related to beta and gamma power.[88] PAF slowing along with increase alpha and theta power oscillations seen in chronic pain states have been shown to reverse with treatment.[89,90] Other abnormalities include reduced beta[91] and increased gamma activity.[92] It is not clear if these changes are seen in all chronic pain states. A study of MEG in multiple sclerosis showed differences in patients with non-neuropathic pain versus those with mixed neuropathic pain.[91]

BRAIN IMAGING IN ANKYLOSING SPONDYLITIS

Cortical gray matter thinning of the primary somatosensory cortex, insular, anterior cingulate and mid-cingulate cortex, prefrontal cortex and supplemental motor area has been shown in a study of patients with AS not on biologic therapy when compared to healthy controls. It also showed increased gray matter volume of the thalamus and putamen. Decreased engagement of the somatosensory cortex and increased engagement of the anterior cingulate cortex correlated with PainDETECT questionnaire scores. All of these findings suggest a mixed picture of pain with neuropathic component of the pain in AS.[19]

A more recent study[93] measured resting-state magnetoencephalography (MEG) spectral density in 45 patients with AS versus 38 age and sex-matched healthy controls. Using PainDETECT, patients with AS were classified as non-neuropathic pain (NNP) and those that had a component of neuropathic pain (NP) in addition to inflammatory back pain. Spectral power was examined in the ascending nociceptive pathway (ANP), DMN, and salience network (SN). Patients with AS compared with healthy controls, showed an increased theta power in the DMN and decreased low-gamma power in the DMN and ANP. However, beta band attenuation or peak alpha slowing was not seen. Patients with NP had increased alpha power in the ANP when compared with healthy controls or patients with NNP. But increased alpha power within ANP was seen in those with reduced BASDAI in the NNP group and increased pain in the mixed-NP group. Thus, high alpha band activity may be a feature of NP while high theta and low gamma activity may be markers of chronic pain.[93]

Fatigue is another common manifestation of active disease in SpA that results in poor concentration and difficulty carrying out tasks due to attention deficit. The attention system consists of 3 distinct networks: the alerting network, the orienting network, and the executive control network. A study comparing 20 patients with AS with 20 age and sex-matched controls subjected to 3T MRI scans and clinical assessment for fatigue, found that fatigue scores negatively correlated to gray matter in the dorsal and ventral attention networks, the somatosensory cortex, and the caudate nucleus.[94] However, they positively correlated to gray matter in the executive control network and putamen. Decreased integrity of the white matter tracts connecting these areas as evidenced by low fractional anisotropy was also seen.

Treatment with TNF not only controls inflammation but also improves pain and fatigue; however, 3T MRI scanning in patients with AS treated with TNF inhibitors show differential effects of TNF inhibitors on pain and fatigue. Although improvement in pain with treatment has been shown to be associated with thinning of the secondary somatosensory cortex as well as motor areas, improvement in fatigue has been shown to be associated with thinning of the insula, primary somatosensory cortex, and superior temporal polysensory areas.[95]

A resting-state fMRI study of 20 patients with AS with chronic pain naïve to anti-TNF therapy versus 20 healthy controls, showed less anti-correlated functional connectivity between the SN and the DMN.[11] The degree of cross-network abnormality correlated with pain as well as disease activity. The posterior cingulate cortex was strongly connected with the SN and weakly connected to the DMN in patients versus healthy controls suggesting that the posterior cingulate cortex may be the hub for altered network interaction.

There has been a growing interest in differences between male and female individuals in terms of pain perception. A recent study that used graph theory with modular analysis and machine learning of resting-state (RS)-fMRI data in 65 patients with AS (45 male and 20 female individuals) versus 155 healthy controls, found sex-specific network topological characteristics in healthy people and those with chronic pain.[96] Higher cross-network connectivity was a feature of those with chronic pain. Higher functional segregation in the mid and subgenual cingulate cortex and lower connectivity in the network with the default mode and fronto-parietal modules was found in female individuals, whereas stronger connectivity with the sensorimotor module was exhibited in male individuals.

PHARMACOTHERAPY OF PAIN IN SPONDYLOARTHRITIS

The medical treatment of SpA usually involves a trial with NSAIDs or Cox-2 inhibitors before considering biologic agents. NSAIDs inhibit cyclooxygenase, which is required for production of prostaglandins, prostacyclins, and thromboxanes. Inhibition of PGE2 that acts on proximal ion channels to sensitize nociceptors, leads to analgesia.[97] Biologic therapy involves blocking important cytokines involved in disease pathogenesis including TNFα, IL-17, and IL-23, resulting in potent immunosuppression. fMRI studies in patients with RA on TNF blockers have been additionally shown to block nociceptive pathways in the thalamus, somatosensory cortex, as well as the limbic system within 24 hours of administration.[98]

Despite all these therapies, there remain 20% to 30% of patients that fail to respond to treatment. Simple analgesics such as acetaminophen or opiate derivatives are not very effective in management of pain in these conditions.[99] With the use of cannabis being legalized around the world, there is a growing interest in this being a potential addition to the list of medications used in this condition. Although self-usage of cannabinoids is reported to be high,[100] evidence of response from randomized clinical trials to prove its efficacy in arthritis is awaited. Given our new understanding of neuropathic nature of pain in some patients with SpA, whether neuropathic medication will prove to be effective in this condition remains to be seen.

SUMMARY

There has been a significant advance in our understanding of pain mechanisms in SpA both through animal models as well as newer modes of neuroimaging. Structural and fMRI show differences in different pain states as well as individuals and newer ways of imaging continue to evolve that may further enhance our understanding of pain. It is now clear that rather than single brain regions, connectivity of different brain networks plays an important role in pain perception and modulation. Important differences between the sexes have been noted both on neuroimaging as well as in animal models that suggest that male and female individuals process pain differently. Although inflammation is an important cause of pain in SpA, evidence now suggests that there may be a neuropathic component of pain in this condition that may need to be addressed in a subgroup of patients.

CLINICS CARE POINTS

- Pain in SpA is multifactorial and includes inflammatory, degenerative, and in some cases neuropathic components.
- The neuroimmune interface allows for a number of immune cells, cytokines, and chemokines to interact with nociceptors as well as cells such as microglia in the nervous system resulting in both peripheral and central sensitization.
- Advances in neuroimaging have illustrated the dynamic nature of connectivity between various brain networks in pain conditions.
- Important differences exist between the sexes in pain pathways, which may have an impact on treatment.

DISCLOSURE

Dr E.M.I. Pathan has received funding for a fellowship from the Spondylitis Program at the University of Toronto. Dr R.D. Inman has no relevant disclosures.

REFERENCES

1. van der Linden S, Valkenburg HA, Cats A. Evaluation of diagnostic criteria for ankylosing spondylitis. A proposal for modification of the New York criteria. Arthritis Rheum 1984;27(4):361–8.
2. Sieper J, Rudwaleit M, Baraliakos X, et al. The Assessment of SpondyloArthritis international Society (ASAS) handbook: a guide to assess spondyloarthritis. Ann Rheum Dis 2009;68(Suppl 2):ii1–44.
3. Kiltz U, Baraliakos X, Regel A, et al. Causes of pain in patients with axial spondyloarthritis. Clin Exp Rheumatol 2017;35(5):S102–7.
4. Maksymowych WP, J.E., Spady B, Russell AS., The Bath Ankylosing Spondylitis Disease Activity Index: Lack of discriminant ability between AS and mechanical low back pain. (Abstract). European League Against Rheumatism Scientific Meeting, Lisbon, Portugal, June 12–15, 2003.
5. de Vlam K, Bokken A. BASDAI is unable to discriminate between inflammatory low back pain and mechanical low back pain [Abstract]. Ann Rheum Dis 2005; 64(suppl III):335.
6. MacKay JW, Aboelmagd S, Gaffney JK. Correlation between clinical and MRI disease activity scores in axial spondyloarthritis. Clin Rheumatol 2015;34: 1633–8.
7. Sieper J, Baraliakos X, Listing J, et al. Persistent reduction of spinal inflammation as assessed by magnetic resonance imaging in patients with ankylosing spondylitis after 2 yrs of treatment with the anti-tumour necrosis factor agent infliximab. Rheumatology (Oxford) 2005;44(12):1525–30.

8. Swinnen TW, Westhovens R, Dankaerts W, et al. Widespread pain in axial spondyloarthritis: clinical importance and gender differences. Arthritis Res Ther 2018;20:156.
9. Macfarlane GJ, Barnish MS, Pathan E, et al. Co-occurrence and characteristics of patients with axial spondyloarthritis who meet criteria for fibromyalgia: results from a UK national register. Arthritis Rheumatol 2017;69(11):2144–50.
10. Shen C-C, Hu L-Y, Yang AC, et al. Risk of psychiatric disorders following ankylosing spondylitis: a nationwide population-based retrospective cohort study. J Rheumatol 2016;43(3):625–31.
11. Hemington KS, Wu Q, Kucyi A, et al. Abnormal cross-network functional connectivity in chronic pain and its association with clinical symptoms. Brain Struct Funct 2016;221(8):4203–19.
12. Gracey E, Yao Y, Green B, et al. Sexual dimorphism in the Th17 signature of ankylosing spondylitis. Arthritis Rheumatol 2016;68(3):679–89.
13. Pedersen SJ, Weber U, Ostergaard M. The diagnostic utility of MRI in spondyloarthritis. Best Pract Res Clin Rheumatol 2012;26(6):751–66.
14. Marzo-Ortega H, McGonagle D, Bennett AN. Magnetic resonance imaging in spondyloarthritis. Curr Opin Rheumatol 2010;22(4):381–7.
15. Blachier M, Coutanceau B, Dougados M, et al. Does the site of magnetic resonance imaging abnormalities match the site of recent-onset inflammatory back pain? The DESIR cohort. Ann Rheum Dis 2013;72:979–85.
16. de Bruin F, ter Horst S, Bloem HL, et al. Prevalence of degenerative changes of the spine on magnetic resonance images and radiographs in patients aged 16–45 years with chronic back pain of short duration in the Spondyloarthritis Caught Early (SPACE) cohort. Rheumatology 2016;55(1):56–65.
17. Lee JS, Lee S, Bang SY, et al. Prevalence and risk factors of anterior atlantoaxial subluxation in ankylosing spondylitis. J Rheumatol 2012;39(12):2321–6.
18. Lo C, Nair KPS, Romanowski CAJ, et al. Horse's tail in bamboo spine: the "cauda equina syndrome in ankylosing spondylitis". Pract Neurol 2014;14(6):418–21.
19. Wu Q, Inman RD, Davis KD. Neuropathic pain in ankylosing spondylitis: a psychophysics and brain imaging study. Arthritis Rheum 2013;65:1494–503.
20. Wach J, Letroublon M-C, Coury F, et al. Fibromyalgia in spondyloarthritis: effect on disease activity assessment in clinical practice. J Rheumatol 2016;43(11):2056–63.
21. Molto A, Etcheto A, Gossec L, et al. Evaluation of the impact of concomitant fibromyalgia on TNF alpha blockers' effectiveness in axial spondyloarthritis: results of a prospective, multicentre study. Ann Rheum Dis 2017;1. annrheumdis-2017e212378.
22. Dubin AE, Patapoutian A. Nociceptors: the sensors of the pain pathway. J Clin Invest 2010;120:3760–72.
23. Gold MS, Gebhart GF. Nociceptor sensitization in pain pathogenesis. Nat Med 2010;16(11):1248–57.
24. Meyer RA, Davis KD, Cohen RH, et al. Mechanically insensitive afferents (MIAs) in cutaneous nerves of monkey. Brain Res 1991;561(2):252–61.
25. Pinho-Ribeiro FA, Verri WA, Chiu IM. Nociceptor sensory neuron–immune interactions in pain and inflammation. Trends Immunol 2017;38(1):5–19.
26. Snider WD, McMahon SB. Tackling pain at the source: New ideas about nociceptors. Neuron 1998;20(4):629–32.
27. Benarroch EE. Ion channels in nociceptors. Neurology 2015;84(11):1153–64.

28. Felson DT. The sources of pain in knee osteoarthritis. Curr Opin Rheumatol 2005;17(5):624–8.
29. Emshoff R, Brandlmaier I, Gerhard S, et al. Magnetic resonance imaging predictors of temporomandibular joint pain. J Am Dent Assoc 2003;134(6):705–14.
30. Hofmann S, Kramer J, Vakil-Adli A, et al. Painful bone marrow edema of the knee: differential diagnosis and therapeutic concepts. Orthop Clin North Am 2004;35(3):321–33.
31. Bennett AN, Rehman A, Hensor EMA, et al. Evaluation of the diagnostic utility of spinal magnetic resonance imaging in axial spondylarthritis. Arthritis Rheum 2009;60(5):1331–41.
32. Lambert RGW, Dhillon SS, Jhangri GS, et al. High prevalence of symptomatic enthesopathy of the shoulder in ankylosing spondylitis: deltoid origin involvement constitutes a hallmark of disease. Arthritis Care Res 2004;51(5):681–90.
33. Cavanaugh JM, Lu Y, Chen C, et al. Pain generation in lumbar and cervical facet joints. J Bone Joint Surg Am 2006;88(Suppl. 2):63–7.
34. Szadek KM, Hoogland PVJM, Zuurmond WWA, et al. Possible nociceptive structures in the sacroiliac joint cartilage: an immunohistochemical study. Clin Anat 2010;23(2):192–8.
35. Rio E, Moseley L, Purdam C, et al. The pain of tendinopathy: physiological or pathophysiological? Sport Med 2014;44(1):9–23.
36. Grace PM, Hutchinson MR, Maier SF, et al. Pathological pain and the neuroimmune interface. Nat Rev Immunol 2014;14(4):217–31.
37. Cunha TM, Verri WA, Schivo IR, et al. Crucial role of neutrophils in the development of mechanical inflammatory hypernociception. J Leukoc Biol 2008;83(4):824–32.
38. Aich A, Afrin LB, Gupta K. Mast cell-mediated mechanisms of nociception. Int J Mol Sci 2015;16(12):29069–92.
39. Kobayashi Y, Kiguchi N, Fukazawa Y, et al. Macrophage-T cell interactions mediate neuropathic pain through the glucocorticoid-induced tumor necrosis factor ligand system. J Biol Chem 2015;290(20):12603–13.
40. Old EA, Nadkarni S, Grist J, et al. Monocytes expressing CX3CR1 orchestrate the development of vincristine-induced pain. J Clin Invest 2014;124(5):2023–36.
41. Kim CF, Moalem-Taylor G. Interleukin-17 contributes to neuroinflammation and neuropathic pain following peripheral nerve injury in mice. J Pain 2011;12(3):370–83.
42. Liu XJ, Zhang Y, Liu T, et al. Nociceptive neurons regulate innate and adaptive immunity and neuropathic pain through MyD88 adapter. Cell Res 2014;24(11):1374–7.
43. Binshtok AM, Wang H, Zimmermann K, et al. Nociceptors are interleukin-1 sensors. J Neurosci 2008;28(52):14062–73.
44. Malsch P, Andratsch M, Vogl C, et al. Deletion of interleukin-6 signal transducer gp130 in small sensory neurons attenuates mechanonociception and downregulates TRPA1 expression. J Neurosci 2014;34(30):9845–56.
45. Fang D, Kong LY, Cai J, et al. Interleukin-6-mediated functional upregulation of TRPV1 receptors in dorsal root ganglion neurons through the activation of JAK/PI3K signaling pathway: roles in the development of bone cancer pain in a rat model. Pain 2015;156(6):1124–44.
46. Jin X, Gereau RW. Acute p38-mediated modulation of tetrodotoxin-resistant sodium channels in mouse sensory neurons by tumor necrosis factor-. J Neurosci 2006;26(1):246–55.

47. Cunha TM, Verri WA, Silva JS, et al. A cascade of cytokines mediates mechanical inflammatory hypernociception in mice. Proc Natl Acad Sci U S A 2005; 102(5):1755–60.
48. Gudes S, Barkai O, Caspi Y, et al. The role of slow and persistent TTX-resistant sodium currents in acute tumor necrosis factor-a-mediated increase in nociceptors excitability. J Neurophysiol 2015;113(2):601–19.
49. Schaible HG. Nociceptive neurons detect cytokines in arthritis. Arthritis Res Ther 2014;16(5):470.
50. Pinto LG, Cunha TM, Vieira SM, et al. IL-17 mediates articular hypernociception in antigeninduced arthritis in mice. Pain 2010;148(2):247–56.
51. Dawes JM, McMahon SB. Chemokines as peripheral pain mediators. Neurosci Lett 2013;557:1–8.
52. Eskander MA, Ruparel S, Green DP, et al. Persistent nociception triggered by nerve growth factor (NGF) is mediated by TRPV1 and oxidative mechanisms. J Neurosci 2015;35(22):8593e603.
53. Lacagnina MJ, Watkins LR, Grace PM. Toll-like receptors and their role in persistent pain. Pharmacol Ther 2017;184:145–58.
54. Cekic C, Linden J. Purinergic regulation of the immune system. Nat Rev Immunol 2016;16(3):177–92.
55. Latremoliere A, Woolf C. Central sensitization: a generator of pain hypersensitivity by central neural plasticity. J Pain 2010;10(9):895–926.
56. Schaible H-G, Ebersberger A, Von Banchet GS. Mechanisms of pain in arthritis. Ann N Y Acad Sci 2002;966:343–54.
57. Bidad K, Gracey E, Hemington KS, et al. Pain in ankylosing spondylitis: a neuro-immune collaboration. Nat Rev Rheumatol 2017;13(7):410–20.
58. Guan Z, Kuhn JA, Wang X, et al. Injured sensory neuron-derived CSF1 induces microglial proliferation and DAP12-dependent pain. Nat Neurosci 2016;19(1): 94–101.
59. Tsuda M, Shigemoto-Mogami Y, Koizumi S, et al. P2X4 receptors induced in spinal microglia gate tactile allodynia after nerve injury. Nature 2003;424(6950): 778–83.
60. Coull JAM, Beggs S, Boudreau D, et al. BDNF from microglia causes the shift in neuronal anion gradient underlying neuropathic pain. Nature 2005;438(7070): 1017–21.
61. Hildebrand ME, Xu J, Dedek A, et al. Potentiation of synaptic GluN2B NMDAR currents by Fyn kinase is gated through BDNF-mediated disinhibition in spinal pain processing. Cell Rep 2016;17(10):2753–65.
62. Sorge RE, Mapplebeck JCS, Rosen S, et al. Different immune cells mediate mechanical pain hypersensitivity in male and female mice. Nat Neurosci 2015; 18(8):1081–3.
63. Park HJ, Stokes JA, Corr M, et al. Toll-like receptor signaling regulates cisplatin induced mechanical allodynia in mice. Cancer Chemother Pharmacol 2014;73: 25–34.
64. Woller SA, Ravula SB, Tucci FC, et al. Systemic TAK-242 prevents intrathecal LPS evoked hyperalgesia in male, but not female mice and prevents delayed allodynia following intraplantar formalin in both male and female mice: The role of TLR4 in the evolution of a persistent pain state. Brain Behav Immun 2016;56:271–80.
65. Stokes JA, Corr M, Yaksh TL. Spinal toll-like receptor signaling and nociceptive processing: regulatory balance between TIRAP and TRIF cascades mediated by TNF and IFN beta. Pain 2013;154:733–42.

66. Fessler MB, Parks JS. Intracellular lipid flux and membrane microdomains as organizing principles in inflammatory cell signaling. J Immunol 2011;187: 1529–35.

67. Schmitz G, Orso E. CD14 signalling in lipid rafts: new ligands and co-receptors. Curr Opin Lipidol 2002;13:513–21.

68. Tall AR, Yvan-Charvet L. Cholesterol, inflammation and innate immunity. Nat Rev Immunol 2015;15:104–16.

69. Woller SA, Choi S-H, An EJ, et al. Inhibition of neuroinflammation by AIBP: Spinal effects upon facilitated pain states. Cell Rep 2018;23(9):2667–77.

70. Gao YJ, Ji RR. Chemokines, neuronal-glial interactions, and central processing of neuropathic pain. Pharmacol Ther 2010;126(1):56–68.

71. Zarpelon AC, Rodrigues FC, Lopes AH, et al. Spinal cord oligodendrocyte-derived alarmin IL-33 mediates neuropathic pain. FASEB J 2016;30(1):54–65.

72. Sorge RE, LaCroix-Fralish ML, Tuttle AH, et al. Spinal cord Toll-like Receptor 4 mediates inflammatory and neuropathic hypersensitivity in male but not female mice. J Neurosci 2011;31(43):15450–4.

73. Hreggvidsdottir HS, Ostberg T, Wahamaa H, et al. The alarmin HMGB1 acts in synergy with endogenous and exogenous danger signals to promote inflammation. J Leukoc Biol 2009;86(3):655–62.

74. Agalave NM, Larsson M, Abdelmoaty S, et al. Spinal HMGB1 induces TLR4-mediated long-lasting hypersensitivity and glial activation and regulates pain-like behavior in experimental arthritis. Pain 2014;155(9):1802–13.

75. Venereau E, Casalgrandi M, Schiraldi M, et al. Mutually exclusive redox forms of HMGB1 promote cell recruitment or proinflammatory cytokine release. J Exp Med 2012;209(9):1519–28.

76. Rudjito R, Agalave NM, Farinotti AB, et al. Sex- and cell-dependent contribution of peripheral high mobility group box 1 and TLR4 in arthritis-induced pain. Pain 2020. https://doi.org/10.1097/j.pain.0000000000002034.

77. Karshikoff B, Lekander M, Soop A, et al. Modality and sex differences in pain sensitivity during human endotoxemia. Brain Behav Immun 2015;46:35–43.

78. Hashmi JA, Davis KD. Deconstructing sex differences in pain sensitivity. Pain 2014;155(1):10–3.

79. Bosma RL, Hemington KS, Davis KD. Using magnetic resonance imaging to visualize the brain in chronic pain. Pain 2017;158(7):1192–3.

80. Davis KD, Moayedi M. Central mechanisms of pain revealed through functional and structural MRI. J Neuroimmune Pharmacol 2013;8(3):518–34.

81. Kucyi A, Davis KD. The dynamic pain connectome. Trends Neurosci 2015;38(2): 86–95.

82. Davis KD, Pope G, Chen J, et al. Cortical thinning in IBS: implications for homeostatic, attention, and pain processing. Neurology 2008;70(2):153–4.

83. Moayedi M, Weissman-Fogel I, Crawley AP, et al. Contribution of chronic pain and neuroticism to abnormal forebrain gray matter in patients with temporomandibular disorder. Neuroimage 2011;55(1):277–86.

84. Seminowicz DA, Wideman TH, Naso L, et al. Effective treatment of chronic low back pain in humans reverses abnormal brain anatomy and function. J Neurosci 2011;31(20):7540–50.

85. Rodriguez-Raecke R, Niemeier A, Ihle K, et al. Brain gray matter decrease in chronic pain is the consequence and not the cause of pain. J Neurosci 2009; 29(44):13746–50.

86. Kucyi A, Davis KD. The neural code for pain: from single-cell electrophysiology to the dynamic pain connectome. Neuroscientist 2017;23(4):397–414.

87. Furman AJ, Meeker TJ, Rietschel JC, et al. Cerebral peak alpha frequency predicts individual differences in pain sensitivity. NeuroImage 2018;167:203–10.
88. May ES, Nickel MM, Ta Dinh S, et al. Prefrontal gamma oscillations reflect ongoing pain intensity in chronic back pain patients. Hum Brain Mapp 2019; 40:293–305.
89. Sarnthein J, Stern J, Aufenberg C, et al. Increased EEG power and slowed dominant frequency in patients with neurogenic pain. Brain 2006;129(1):55–64.
90. Stern J, Jeanmonod D, Sarnthein J. Persistent EEG overactivation in the cortical pain matrix of neurogenic pain patients. NeuroImage 2006;31(2):721–31.
91. Kim J, Bosma R, Hemington KS, et al. Neuropathic pain and pain interference are linked to alpha-band slowing and reduced beta-band magnetoencephalography activity within the dynamic pain connectome in patients with multiple sclerosis. Pain 2019;160(1):187–97.
92. Lim M, Kim JS, Kim DJ, et al. Increased low-and high-frequency oscillatory activity in the prefrontal cortex of fibromyalgia patients. Front Hum Neurosci 2016; 10:111.
93. Kisler LB, Kim JA, Hemington KS, et al. Abnormal alpha band power in the dynamic pain connectome is a marker of chronic pain with a neuropathic component. NeuroImage Clin 2020;26:102241.
94. Wu Q, Inman RD, Davis KD. Fatigue in ankylosing spondylitis is associated with the brain networks of sensory salience and attention. Arthritis Rheum 2014; 66(2).295–303.
95. Wu Q, Inman RD, Davis KD. Tumor necrosis factor inhibitor therapy in ankylosing spondylitis. Pain 2015;156(2):297–304.
96. Fauchon C, Meunier D, Rogachov A, et al. Sex differences in brain modular organization in chronic pain. Pain 2020. https://doi.org/10.1097/j.pain.0000000000002104.
97. Ferreira SH. Prostaglandins, aspirin-like drugs and analgesia. Nat New Biol 1972;240(102):200–3.
98. Hess A, Axmann R, Rech J, et al. Blockade of TNF-a rapidly inhibits pain responses in the central nervous system. Proc Natl Acad Sci U S A 2011; 108(9):3731–6.
99. Van Der Heijde D, Ramiro S, Landewe R, et al. 2016 update of the ASAS-EULAR management recommendations for axial spondyloarthritis. Ann Rheum Dis 2017;76(6):978–91.
100. Lucas P, Walsh Z. Medical cannabis access, use, and substitution for prescription opioids and other substances: a survey of authorized medical cannabis patients. Int J Drug Policy 2017;42:30–5.

The Categorization of Pain in Systemic Lupus Erythematosus

David S. Pisetsky, MD, PhD[a,b,*], Amanda M. Eudy, PhD[a],
Megan E.B. Clowse, MD[a], Jennifer L. Rogers, MD[a]

KEYWORDS

- Systemic lupus erythematosus • Autoimmunity • Pain • Arthritis • Fibromyalgia
- Quality of life • Depression • Immunosuppression

KEY POINTS

- Lupus is a systemic autoimmune disease characterized by multiple sources of pain.
- Arthritis is the most common form of musculoskeletal pain in lupus.
- Symptoms in lupus can be divided into 2 categories called type 1 and type 2.
- Type 1 and type 2 symptoms can differ in response to immunosuppressive agents.
- Fibromyalgia can cause widespread pain in lupus.

Systemic lupus erythematosus (SLE) is a prototypic autoimmune disease characterized by immunologic disturbances and diverse symptoms that vary in pattern and severity among patients.[1,2] These disturbances are highly interconnected and underlie many of the clinical and laboratory findings of SLE, including the prominent expression of antinuclear antibodies.[3] In view of the unequivocal evidence of immune cell disturbance in SLE, investigators have tended to view disease pathogenesis as well as disease manifestations primarily in terms of immunology. Because current technologies are providing a more detailed picture of cellular abnormalities than ever before possible, investigative interest in this area has surged.[4]

Although characterizing immune abnormalities is eminently appropriate for an autoimmune disease, such a focus may not adequately incorporate the patient perspective and the wide range of symptoms of SLE that can impact quality of life. SLE is a disease of tissue inflammation and injury. It is also a very painful disease in which pain can dominate the lived experience of the patient.[5] Furthermore, pain in SLE can occur in

[a] Division of Rheumatology and Immunology, Duke University Medical Center, Durham, NC, USA; [b] Medical Research Service, Durham Veterans Administration Medical Center, Durham, NC, USA
* Corresponding author. Duke University Medical Center, Medical Research Service, Durham VA Medical Center, Durham, NC 27710.
E-mail address: david.pisetsky@duke.edu

Rheum Dis Clin N Am 47 (2021) 215–228
https://doi.org/10.1016/j.rdc.2020.12.004
0889-857X/21/© 2020 Elsevier Inc. All rights reserved.

rheumatic.theclinics.com

the context of other symptoms such as fatigue, which can impair quality of life beyond the consequences of inflammatory injury of the tissues.[6–9]

For the patient, pain is often the symptom that brings them to the physician, with pain relief the proximate goal of therapy. For the physician or other provider evaluating such a patient, the challenge is to understand the origin of the pain, assess its relationship to inflammation, and develop a treatment plan to decrease its impact. In the treatment of SLE, pain management is a particular challenge because the relationship of pain to inflammation is often obscure, with immunomodulatory therapy frequently unsuccessful. As a result, patients may experience inadequate symptom relief, leading to dissatisfaction with the medical encounter. Discordancy between patients and providers in the assessment of the basis of symptoms can, unfortunately, complicate communication and prevent the establishment of an effective therapeutic relationship.[10–12]

In our unit, we have been exploring a new approach to the management of pain in SLE that we hope will improve overall patient care. This approach is based on the division of signs and symptoms of SLE into 2 broad categories that are termed type 1 and type 2; in view of their temporal variation, both types can be assessed at the time of each medical visit.[13,14] Type 1 manifestations are the classic signs and symptoms of SLE that are, in general, immunologically mediated. These manifestations include nephritis, inflammatory arthritis, rash and serositis. Type 2 manifestations include pain (especially fibromyalgia), fatigue, depression, sleep disturbance, and perceived cognitive dysfunction.

In this article, we review the manifestations of SLE that are painful and then discuss in greater detail the application of the type 1 and type 2 categorization to patient care. As this discussion proceeds, it is important to note that we consider both type 1 and type 2 symptoms as manifestations of the underlying disease pathogenesis in SLE, even if the link between certain symptoms and immune cell abnormalities may be obscure at the present time.

MUSCULOSKELETAL PAIN

Table 1 lists the cause of pain attributable to the musculoskeletal system. These manifestations encompass both inflammation and damage as well as symptoms that would be categorized as type 2 symptoms.

Arthritis

The importance of arthritis as a manifestation of SLE has grown, especially in the setting of clinical trials for new agents to treat this disease. In the development path, the usual first step is the assessment of the ensemble of manifestations known

Table 1 Sources of musculoskeletal pain	
Condition	**Mechanism**
Arthritis	Activity
Myositis	Activity
Avascular necrosis	Damage
Fracture	Damage
Osteoarthritis	?
Fibromyalgia	Type 2

as nonrenal SLE, which primarily involve musculoskeletal and mucocutaneous manifestations.[15] Unlike nephritis, which has been extensively investigated in animal
models of disease and has a well-validated disease mechanism (ie, immune complex
deposition), arthritis and related musculoskeletal manifestations have lacked a clear
model or experimental framework to elucidate mechanisms.

According to classical concepts of arthritis in SLE, patients can display 3 distinct
patterns of joint involvement: (1) a symmetric polyarthritis involving primarily the small
joints, with prominent involvement of the fingers and wrists, (2) a nonerosive deforming
arthritis, termed Jaccoud's arthropathy, characterized by reducible ulnar deviation
and swan neck deformities owing to ligamentous and joint capsule laxity, and (3) an
overlap between SLE and rheumatoid arthritis (RA) that is characterized by serologic
disturbances similar to those of RA (ie, anti–cyclic citrullinated peptide and rheumatoid
factor).[16,17] This overlap condition has sometimes been called "rhupus." **Box 1** presents definitions of joint involvement in SLE used to measure for assessing classification or disease activity.[18–20]

According to the older literature, the small joint form of arthritis is marked by pain out
of proportion to the findings on physical examination and, although joint tenderness
can be elicited, swelling has been considered to be mild. Because plain radiographs
do not show evidence of erosion, patient reports of pain and tenderness have repre-
sented the most substantial evidence of synovitis.

More recent studies are redefining the nature of arthritis in SLE, positing greater sim-
ilarity to RA than historically thought. One possibility for the changing perspective relates to changes in the nature of synovitis in RA, which is the prime example of an
inflammatory arthritis with which others are compared. As many clinicians can attest,
RA now seems to be a less severe condition than before; this situation
perhaps reflects earlier recognition and treatment with more effective disease-
modifying antirheumatic drugs.[21] In RA at present, synovitis seems to be less prominent and both erosion and deformity are markedly attenuated. In the care of patients
with RA, clinicians have adapted to a picture of a much less severe disease, interpret-
ing lesser degrees of synovitis as, nevertheless, clinically significant.

Now that clinicians are accustomed to assessing more limited joint findings as evidence of active RA, they are perhaps paying more attention to synovitis in SLE. As
such, the same metrics used to assess disease activity in RA (eg, DAS28) are being
applied to SLE.[22–24] Indeed, studies have demonstrated that, in SLE, both joint tenderness and swelling can involve numerous joints in seeming contradiction to previous
ideas that arthritis in SLE is characterized by tenderness out of proportion to swelling.

Along with a change in the findings noted on the physical examination, new approaches to imaging have documented more objective findings of lupus arthritis.[25–28]

Box 1
Definitions of Arthritis or Joint Involvement in SLE

Systemic Lupus International Collaborating Clinics Criteria for Disease Classification
   Synovitis involving 2 or more joints, characterized by swelling or effusion OR tenderness of 2
   more joints and 30 minutes of morning stiffness

2019 American College of Rheumatology–European League Against Rheumatism Criteria for
Disease Classification
   EITHER (1) synovitis involving 2 or more joints characterized by swelling or effusion OR (2)
   tenderness in 2 or more joints and at least 30 minutes of morning stiffness

Systemic Lupus Erythematosus Disease Activity Index
   More than 2 joints with pain and signs of inflammation (ie, tenderness, swelling, or effusion)

Ultrasound imaging of joints in patients with SLE can demonstrate synovitis, with most studies concentrating on the fingers and wrists. In addition, ultrasound examination can show a prominent tenosynovitis, a finding that may be relevant to the development of deformity.

Even though SLE arthritis has been considered nonerosive (with the exception of the rhupus overlap), imaging by both ultrasound examination and MRI can show bone marrow changes. Changes of this kind are common in studies of RA and are thought to represent an early stage in the erosive process; nevertheless, it is possible that these changes indicate inflammation or edema in the bone marrow, which may not progress to actual cortical breaks demonstrable on plain films.

The advances in imaging raise important questions concerning the best approach to assessing pain in arthritis in the clinical setting and developing a treatment strategy analogous to treat-to-target strategies in RA.[29] Whereas in RA the goal of treatment is to decrease pain and retard erosion and deformity, the goal in SLE is primarily to decrease pain because erosion seems uncommon or at least different in kind from that in RA. In view of recent studies showing that measures such as the DAS28 are applicable to RA, it seems to be reasonable to base treatment decisions on a tender and swollen joint count, although symptoms and imaging may not be directly related. In SLE, the effects of certain cytokines may decrease levels of C-reactive protein, however, making it less reliable as a measure of inflammation.[30]

Once a framework for assessing inflammatory arthritis in SLE is established in the routine care setting, then the usual agents to treat this condition include hydroxychloroquine, methotrexate, nonsteroidal anti-inflammatory drugs, and glucocorticoids. Because a drug like belimumab is approved for nonrenal manifestations of active, autoantibody-positive SLE, it is often used for the treatment of arthritis because studies have indicated an effect on musculoskeletal manifestations as a part of conventional measures of disease activity.[31]

Myositis

Whereas myalgia is not an uncommon source of pain in SLE, some patients develop signs and symptoms of an inflammatory myopathy.[32,33] In these patients, muscle pain and tenderness can accompany weakness. The frequency of myositis in SLE varies widely depending on the case definition and, for example, the requirement for elevation of creatinine phosphokinase for diagnosis. One study suggested that myositis in SLE is marked by elevation of levels of aldolase rather than creatinine phosphokinase.[32] An evaluation for myositis would depend on findings of weakness, although this assessment can be complicated by the presence of a steroid myopathy or deconditioning.

Avascular Necrosis

In contrast with inflammatory arthritis, which is a sign of disease activity, avascular necrosis (AVN) is a sign of damage and a source of intense pain.[34–36] This condition can affect multiple joints, although large joints such as the knees and the hips are the most common. The etiology of AVN in SLE seems to be complex, with contributions from underlying immunologic and hematologic disturbances as well as the effects of glucocorticoids. Whatever the exact interplay of these disturbances are, AVN results from ischemia to bone with subsequent death and collapse.

Clotting disturbances, including the antiphospholipid antibody syndrome, are among the potential factors contributing to the development of AVN in SLE, but are difficult to assess because of the concurrent use of glucocorticoids.

Among its many actions that lead to damage in SLE, glucocorticoids are clearly associated with the development of AVN. Given the diverse manner in which glucocorticoids are prescribed in SLE, determining the relationship of dose to the development of AVN is difficult. Thus, it is not clear whether the major determinant of AVN is total glucocorticoid dose, average glucocorticoid dose, or highest glucocorticoid dose.

In general, the diagnosis of AVN is made on the basis of symptoms of pain, with plain films demonstrating various stages of radiographic progression. MRI is also a useful modality in evaluating pain in patients suspected of AVN; furthermore, it can show changes in regions that may not be symptomatic. As in the case of AVN in patients with other conditions, therapy includes surgery with core decompression and bone grafting as well as total joint replacement.[37] AVN is one of the most frequent reasons for total joint replacement for patients and is one setting when more pain relief can be achieved decisively.

Fracture

Osteoporotic fracture is another source of musculoskeletal pain in SLE that seems to be complex in etiology.[38–40] The most common locations are the hips, vertebrae and humerus. Although glucocorticoid-induced osteoporosis is a main etiology, other factors can lead to bone loss. These factors include vitamin D deficiency from sun avoidance, immobility, lack of weight-bearing exercise, lupus nephritis, disease duration, prior history of fracture, and generalized disease activity. Bone loss is a feature of a proinflammatory state, with agents that can decrease inflammation potentially able to retard bone loss. Glucocorticoids, however, have their own direct effects on bone, leading to glucocorticoid-induced osteoporosis.

As in the case of AVN, the occurrence of fracture provides a strong impetus to limit glucocorticoid use by substitution of other agents without this complication. The prevention of glucocorticoid-induced osteoporosis by antiresorptive therapy can be an important strategy to decrease fracture risk. In SLE, however, the use of agents such as bisphosphonates must take into account patient age and child-bearing potential because bisphosphonates are in pregnancy class C.

Osteoarthritis

With better therapy for SLE, the overall outcomes of patients with SLE have improved. Patients are living longer and, not surprisingly, osteoarthritis can occur, providing another source of pain in those patients with longstanding disease.[41] Although precise data on the frequency of osteoarthritis are difficult to obtain, the frequency of total joint replacement in patients with SLE allows inference on the development of this condition.[37] Unlike other musculoskeletal manifestations of SLE, osteoarthritis is difficult to categorize as either activity or damage.

Fibromyalgia

Of the various sources of musculoskeletal pain in SLE, fibromyalgia is among the most common.[42,43] Fibromyalgia is a chronic, painful condition in which disturbances in neuropsychological function and sensitization lead to pain amplification.[44–46] Widespread body pain is the hallmark, with tender points providing support for a role of pain amplification. Rather than calling fibromyalgia a disease or state, "fibromyalgianess" can be conceptualized as a trait that can also condition the perception of other painful conditions.

Despite causing significant distress, fibromyalgia does not fit well as either activity or damage; as such, fibromyalgia, along with other symptoms, may not receive the same efforts at treatment and prevention as those disease manifestations that are more clearly immunologically mediated. As many studies show, fibromyalgia is frequent in SLE and, although the assessment of fibromyalgia can be difficult, the occurrence of this condition in SLE is far greater than the general population.[42,43] The coexistence of fibromyalgia and arthritis occurs with other inflammatory diseases, such as spondyloarthritis, raising the possibility that it may be a consequence of localized pain, inflammation, or stress.[47]

In the context of other sources of musculoskeletal pain, awareness of fibromyalgia is important because it can allow for an interpretation of the findings of tenderness in the absence of swelling or high pain reports in patients with peripheral arthritis whose joint examination shows little or no evidence of synovitis.

NEUROPSYCHOLOGICAL SOURCES OF PAIN
Headache

Among the sources of pain in SLE, headache is notable because it is a criterion for disease activity in the Systemic Lupus Erythematosus Disease Activity Index.[18] Despite this standing, the nature of headache in SLE is unclear.[48–51] Furthermore, it is unclear whether the frequency of headache in SLE is any greater than the general population, recognizing that the frequency of headache in the population depends on age and sex. One of the reasons for uncertainty about headache as a manifestation of SLE relates to the definition of headache by various organizations. For example, in the Systemic Lupus Erythematosus Disease Activity Index, lupus headache is defined as "severe persistent headache, may be migrainous, but must be nonresponsive to narcotic analgesia." In contrast, the International Headache Society provides a different categorization of headaches, in general, denoting tension headache as well as migraine headache with or without aura as common forms of headache in the population. Using the International Headache Society criteria, most headaches in SLE can be readily characterized in the usual symptom categories. Although such considerations do not exclude the existence of a distinct headache associated with disease activity, it seems reasonable to manage headache according to the usual approach for the general population.

Small Fiber Neuropathy

As a systemic disease, SLE has protean manifestations that occur with widely varying frequency. Although not included in the 19 neuropsychiatric syndromes as defined by the American College of Rheumatology,[52] small fiber neuropathy can lead to diffuse pain, burning, tingling, numbness, and changes in thermal sensation. Diagnosis is confirmed by skin biopsy, demonstrating a decreased intraepidermal nerve fiber density.[53,54] Treatment involves the usual medications for neuropathic pain; there are data supporting the use of intravenous IgG.[55]

SEROSITIS

Pericarditis and pleuritis can both present with sudden and severe pain along with signs of inflammation and demonstration of effusions by either chest radiographs or ultrasound examination.[56,57] In contrast with other sources of pain that have been discussed, serositis represents an acute situation that demands prompt diagnosis and treatment, including the exclusion of infection. Depending on the severity of these conditions, therapy may involve nonsteroidal anti-inflammatory drugs, colchicine, or glucocorticoids.

For some patients with SLE, chest pain may occur in the absence of other evidence of pleuritis or pericarditis. These patients are often treated with anti-inflammatory agents, even if the evidence for inflammation is scant. In this setting, there is concern about overtreatment with glucocorticoids.

Peritonitis can also present a diagnostic challenge, because abdominal pain can signal a wide variety of serious visceral ailments, including emergent problems such as a perforation or bowel infarction. Therefore, the diagnostic workup must be detailed, with concern for conditions that need surgical attention.

OTHER CONDITIONS

Patients with SLE can develop other sources of pain that may arise from immunologic disturbances (eg, vasculitis leading to infarction), the effects of drugs (eg, pancreatitis or esophagitis from glucocorticoids or nonsteroidal anti-inflammatory drugs), or coincidence. Not everything that occurs in patients with SLE need be attributed to that disease. For the more acute painful conditions, the workup has to be sufficient to exclude problems that would demand therapies other than anti-inflammatory or immunosuppressive agents.

SYMPTOM CATEGORIZATION
The Type 1–Type 2 Paradigm

According to current thinking about SLE pathogenesis, clinical manifestations can, in general, be divided into 2 broad categories: activity and damage.[18,58–60] This categorization suffices for manifestations such as nephritis, where biopsies can show signs of inflammation (activity) or scarring and fibrosis (damage). Among the main complaints of patients with SLE are a series of symptoms that can be difficult to bin into these 2 categories. These symptoms include fatigue, pain, depression, sleep disturbance, and perceived cognitive dysfunction. The origin of these symptoms is often obscure and seemingly lacks a relationship to conventional measures of disease activity. It is perhaps surprising that one of the main complaints of patients (ie, fatigue) does not signify disease activity; it also does not signify damage.

Our clinic has proposed a different scheme for symptom categorization in SLE that does not rely on the simple dichotomy of activity and damage. Rather, we have proposed that symptoms of SLE activity can be divided into 2 main categories or bins that are simply called type 1 and type 2 symptoms. As noted elsewhere in this article, type 1 symptoms are the classical signs and symptoms of SLE that can be clearly ascribed to inflammation and autoreactivity. Nephritis is at the top of the list. There are excellent biomarkers for nephritis in terms of renal function, tissue pathology, and serology. Rash is another example of type 1 manifestation where an immune mechanism can be established. Importantly, some type 1 manifestations are asymptomatic and patients may be unaware of serious renal disease.

In contrast with the type 1 manifestations, type 2 manifestations are all symptomatic, with the magnitude, persistence, and pervasiveness of these symptoms often dominating the patient experience of this illness. For type 2 symptoms, it can be difficult to establish a link between the symptoms, on the one hand, and inflammation and autoreactivity, on the other hand. Furthermore, by their nature, some of these symptoms can be multifactorial in origin. For example, depression can result from the burden of chronic illness, unrelenting pain, loss of employment and, disability.

Although type 2 symptoms may not show obvious links to inflammation, they may, nevertheless, result from immune activity. Thus, cytokines can act as mediators in the central and peripheral nervous system and there is substantial evidence that proinflammatory cytokines contribute to symptoms of pain, fatigue, and depression. Clinical trials have shown efficacy of tumor necrosis factor-α blockers in ordinary depression although the benefits may be greatest in those with elevation of C-reactive protein.[61] Similarly, tumor necrosis factor-α blockers have ameliorated depression in patients with psoriasis.[62]

As a group, pain, fatigue, depression, and cognitive dysfunction often track together, especially in patients with chronic inflammatory disease. In this setting, the array of symptoms is analogous to so-called sickness behavior that describes the symptoms that accompany acute inflammatory and infectious illnesses.[63] These symptoms are part of an overall host response that can influence energy metabolism to shift nutrients to fuel an immune response to overcome infection. The infected (or inflamed) person becomes tired and sedentary, showing weakness, lassitude, and pain to deter more strenuous activities that would be energetically demanding. Although this program may have evolved for acute host defense and be physiologic or protective in the acute setting, it can be replayed in the setting of a chronic inflammatory disease and become pathologic.[64,65]

The division of symptoms into type 1 and type 2 categories does not mean that type 2 symptoms are totally or substantially independent of inflammatory mediators. Rather, the division signifies that the 2 types of symptoms can occur independently, with type 2 symptoms often dissociated from flares of SLE and increases in measures of disease. Importantly, the division indicates that therapies necessary to decrease type 1 and type 2 symptoms may be different and that immunosuppressive agents for type 1 symptoms may not attenuate type 2 symptoms. As manifestations of SLE, type 2 symptoms demand their own therapies as part of a more comprehensive treatment program, even if these therapies are seemingly unrelated to the immune system. In contrast, data from clinical trials indicate an effect of belimumab on fatigue.[66] Importantly, patients can have both type 1 and type 2 manifestations in varying extents (**Fig. 1**).

The Rationale of the Type 1–Type 2 System for the Management of Pain

The type 1–type 2 categorization is a theoretic construct whose goal is to elucidate better the origin of symptoms, including pain, in patients with SLE, to enhance patient–provider communication, and to improve patient quality of life by addressing the full gamut of patient symptoms. In this construct, the totality of symptoms that the patient reports constitute their "lupus" because that is how patients understand their disease. Unlike investigators or practitioners, patients do not engage in attribution because they want relief from the full range of symptoms.

As shown by many studies, there is frequent discordance between patients and providers in the assessment of disease activity or severity, contributing to problems in communication and patient dissatisfaction.[10–12] We believe that this discordance relates in part to the relative weight that patients and providers place on different disease manifestations. Whereas providers may focus on type 1 manifestations to form an assessment of disease activity, patients may focus on type 2 manifestations because these manifestations, by their nature, are very symptomatic. In terms of pain, the provider may perform a joint examination and find minimal tenderness, concluding that

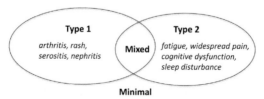

Fig. 1. The figure illustrates the relationship between type 1 and type 2 manifestations, demonstrating the overlap between the 2 categories. Some patients may report neither type 1 nor type 2 symptoms and can be considered to have minimal SLE.

arthritis is inactive. In contrast, the patient may be experiencing widespread pain, with fibromyalgia underlying the patient assessment that the disease is very active.

Regarding that both type 1 and type 2 symptoms are essential elements in disease has important implications for therapy. First, patient–provider communication can be enhanced by validating the symptoms that patients report (eg, fibromyalgia) are, indeed, a part of their condition, requiring evaluation and treatment. Second, by recognizing that type 1 and type 2 symptoms may have distinct origins, even in the same patient, the provider can choose therapy more appropriately, expanding beyond the base of immunosuppressive agents. A more thoughtful approach to therapy based on the type 1–type 2 categorization can limit the use of corticosteroids for problems that are not primarily inflammatory in origin.

Just as the categorization of symptoms into type 1 and type 2 bins may decrease the use of immunosuppressive agents, it may also increase the use of other classes of drugs related to fibromyalgia or depression. As a study from our clinic has found, depression in SLE is frequently undertreated because it is not clearly a manifestation of neuropsychologic lupus and can be complex in its etiology.[67] By incorporating depression in the type 1–type 2 paradigm, the issue of attribution becomes less pressing and a more satisfactory treatment plan can be developed to include exercise and stress reduction, for example.

The Application of the Type 1–Type 2 Paradigm to Treatment

In our clinic, we have begun more formal application of the type 1–type 2 system in routine care and are constructing a research platform to investigate many issues that flow from this type of a more holistic patient approach.

At present, there are a variety of measures for type 1 disease that range from patient reports and surveys for disease activity to laboratory testing to sophisticated molecular analyses to interrogate immune response. The measures for type 2 disease are also many but, in general, these are patient reports that have been developed for other settings (eg, depression, fatigue) not necessarily related to lupus. The use of measures for type 2 manifestation at this time must be borrowed from other conditions, pending the development of measures that are more specific for SLE.

For our initial operationalization of care according to the type 1–type 2 system, we have used the Systemic Lupus Erythematosus Disease Activity Index for type 1 disease activity. For type 2 symptoms, we have used the 2011 American College of Rheumatology fibromyalgia criteria, considering a widespread index score of 7 or higher and a symptom severity score 5 or higher, or a widespread pain index of 3 or higher and a symptom severity score of 9 or higher as indicative of type 2 disease. We chose this measure because it does relate to pain, a major type 2 symptom, and is consistent with studies indicating the frequency of fibromyalgia in SLE.[42,43] In using this scale, we are considering fibromyalgia as a trait that can be of varying intensity or severity. In our use, the total fibromyalgia severity score (a sum of the widespread pain index and the symptom severity score) can provide a measure of "fibromyalgianess" that can lead to symptoms itself (ie, widespread body pain) or color or condition the reporting of other symptoms (eg, hair loss, chest pain).

Our first study showed how the incorporation of assessment for both type 1 and type 2 can lead to a new and hopefully more informative categorization of patients that goes beyond the more classic activity–damage dichotomy.[14] The use of 2 measures allows the delineation of 4 patient groups as indicated in **Box 2**, although more subdivisions are possible.

Using the type 1 and type 2 categorization, we found that 20% of patients can be categorized as having high type 2 SLE activity. As a group, patients with type 2 SLE

Box 2
Categorization of symptoms in SLE

Type 1 SLE: Active SLE without meeting fibromyalgia or polysymptomatic distress criteria

Type 2 SLE: Inactive SLE meeting fibromyalgia or polysymptomatic distress criteria

Mixed SLE: Active SLE meeting fibromyalgia or polysymptomatic distress criteria

Minimal SLE: Inactive SLE without meeting fibromyalgia of polysymptomatic distress criteria.

In our studies, we have identified type 2 SLE using either criteria for fibromyalgia or polysymptomatic distress.

---

activity had more severe self-reported lupus activity and higher rates of lupus flares than those without type 2 activity. Moreover, we found that patients with type 2 SLE reported a higher frequency of many symptoms, including fatigue, muscle pain, forgetfulness, and headache; they also reported symptoms that are potentially inflammatory in origin. Although synovitis was not documented on examination in patients with type 2 SLE, the frequency of self-reported joint swelling was similar between patients with type 1 and type 2 SLE.

Our understanding and application of the type 1 and type 2 SLE model are in evolution with, for example, a preliminary cluster analysis indicating there may be more than 4 categories of type 1 and type 2 SLE symptoms including those with fatigue predominant type 2. Moreover, we have found that the severity of type 1 and type 2 activity can fluctuate between visits, even resulting in a change in category.[68]

SUMMARY

Pain in SLE is a major symptom of patients and can result from a wide variety of processes. Although some types of pain may result from immunologic mechanisms associated with inflammation and autoreactivity, other types of pain seem to reflect central mechanisms. To understand and treat pain more effectively, we have proposed a new system to divide symptoms of lupus into 2 broad categories, both of which are intrinsic features of disease. Hopefully, this categorization will promote better communication between patients and providers as well as represent a more effective framework for treating one of the most persistent, severe, and disabling manifestations of SLE.

CLINICS CARE POINTS

- The approach to therapy of patients with SLE can be based on division of the manifestations into 2 categories.
- Inflammatory manifestations (type 1) are related to disease activity and include arthritis and nephritis. These manifestations can respond to immunomodulatory agents.
- Noninflammatory manifestations (type 2) include widespread pain, fatigue, depression, and sleep disturbance. These manifestations do not generally respond to immunomodulatory agents and need other treatments.
- Type 2 manifestations represent some of the common and persistent symptoms of SLE and can impact quality of life.
- Type 1 manifestations can be assessed by the Systemic Lupus Erythematosus Disease Activity Index while type 2 manifestations can be assessed by instruments for fibromyalgia and fatigue.

ACKNOWLEDGMENTS

A.M. Eudy acknowledges the grant support of NIH NCATS 1KL2TR002554.

DISCLOSURE

The authors have no conflicts of interest to disclose.

REFERENCES

1. Lisnevskaia L, Murphy G, Isenberg D. Systemic lupus erythematosus. Lancet 2014;384:1878–88.
2. Kaul A, Gordon C, Crow MK, et al. Systemic lupus erythematosus. Nat Rev Dis Primers 2016;2:16039.
3. Tsokos GC. Systemic lupus erythematosus. N Engl J Med 2011;365:2110–21.
4. Catalina MD, Owen KA, Labonte AC, et al. The pathogenesis of systemic lupus erythematosus: harnessing big data to understand the molecular basis of lupus. J Autoimmun 2020;110:102359.
5. Waldheim E, Elkan AC, Bergman S, et al. Extent and characteristics of self-reported pain in patients with systemic lupus erythematosus. Lupus 2013;22: 136–43.
6. Yazdany J, Yelin E. Health-related quality of life and employment among persons with systemic lupus erythematosus. Rheum Dis Clin North Am 2010;36:15–32, vii.
7. Waldheim E, Elkan AC, Pettersson S, et al. Health-related quality of life, fatigue and mood in patients with SLE and high levels of pain compared to controls and patients with low levels of pain. Lupus 2013;22:1118–27.
8. Fonseca R, Bernardes M, Terroso G, et al. Silent burdens in disease: fatigue and depression in SLE. Autoimmune Dis 2014;2014:790724.
9. Azizoddin DR, Gandhi N, Weinberg S, et al. Fatigue in systemic lupus: the role of disease activity and its correlates. Lupus 2019;28:163–73.
10. Alarcon GS, McGwin G Jr, Brooks K, et al. Systemic lupus erythematosus in three ethnic groups. XI. Sources of discrepancy in perception of disease activity: a comparison of physician and patient visual analog scale scores. Arthritis Rheum 2002;47:408–13.
11. Neville C, Clarke AE, Joseph L, et al. Learning from discordance in patient and physician global assessments of systemic lupus erythematosus disease activity. J Rheumatol 2000;27:675–9.
12. Golder V, Ooi JJY, Antony AS, et al. Discordance of patient and physician health status concerns in systemic lupus erythematosus. Lupus 2018;27:501–6.
13. Pisetsky DS, Clowse MEB, Criscione-Schreiber LG, et al. A novel system to categorize the symptoms of systemic lupus erythematosus. Arthritis Care Res 2019; 71:735–41.
14. Rogers JL, Eudy AM, Pisetsky D, et al. Utilizing clinical characteristics and patient-reported outcome measures to categorize lupus subtypes. Arthritis Care Res 2020. https://doi.org/10.1002/acr.24135.
15. Dall'Era M, Wofsy D. Clinical trial design in systemic lupus erythematosus. Curr Opin Rheumatol 2006;18:476–80.
16. Grossman JM. Lupus arthritis. Best Pract Res Clin Rheumatol 2009;23:495–506.
17. Ceccarelli F, Perricone C, Cipriano E, et al. Joint involvement in systemic lupus erythematosus: from pathogenesis to clinical assessment. Semin Arthritis Rheum 2017;47:53–64.

18. Bombardier C, Gladman DD, Urowitz MB, et al. Derivation of the SLEDAI. A disease activity index for lupus patients. The Committee on Prognosis Studies in SLE. Arthritis Rheum 1992;35:630–40.
19. Petri M, Orbai AM, Alarcon GS, et al. Derivation and validation of the Systemic Lupus International Collaborating Clinics classification criteria for systemic lupus erythematosus. Arthritis Rheum 2012;64:2677–86.
20. Aringer M, Costenbader K, Daikh D, et al. 2019 European League Against Rheumatism/American College of Rheumatology Classification Criteria for Systemic Lupus Erythematosus. Arthritis Rheumatol 2019;71:1400–12.
21. Aletaha D, Smolen JS. Diagnosis and management of rheumatoid arthritis: a review. JAMA 2018;320:1360–72.
22. Castrejón I, Yazici Y, Pincus T. Patient self-report RADAI (Rheumatoid Arthritis Disease Activity Index) joint counts on an MDHAQ (Multidimensional Health Assessment Questionnaire) in usual care of consecutive patients with rheumatic diseases other than rheumatoid arthritis. Arthritis Care Res 2013;65:288–93.
23. Ceccarelli F, Perricone C, Massaro L, et al. The role of disease activity score 28 in the evaluation of articular involvement in systemic lupus erythematosus. ScientificWorldJournal 2014;2014:236842.
24. Cipriano E, Ceccarelli F, Massaro L, et al. Joint involvement in patients affected by systemic lupus erythematosus: application of the swollen to tender joint count ratio. Reumatismo 2015;67:62–7.
25. Tani C, D'Aniello D, Possemato N, et al. MRI pattern of arthritis in systemic lupus erythematosus: a comparative study with rheumatoid arthritis and healthy subjects. Skeletal Radiol 2015;44:261–6.
26. Piga M, Saba L, Gabba A, et al. Ultrasonographic assessment of bone erosions in the different subtypes of systemic lupus erythematosus arthritis: comparison with computed tomography. Arthritis Res Ther 2016;18:222.
27. Torrente-Segarra V, Monte TCS, Corominas H. Musculoskeletal involvement and ultrasonography update in systemic lupus erythematosus: new insights and review. Eur J Rheumatol 2018;5:127–30.
28. Zollars ES, Hyer M, Wolf B, et al. Measuring lupus arthritis activity using contrasted high-field MRI. Associations with clinical measures of disease activity and novel patterns of disease. Lupus Sci Med 2018;5:e000264.
29. Smolen JS, Breedveld FC, Burmester GR, et al. Treating rheumatoid arthritis to target: 2014 update of the recommendations of an international task force. Ann Rheum Dis 2016;75:3–15.
30. Enocsson H, Sjowall C, Skogh T, et al. Interferon-alpha mediates suppression of C-reactive protein: explanation for muted C-reactive protein response in lupus flares? Arthritis Rheum 2009;60:3755–60.
31. Manzi S, Sánchez-Guerrero J, Merrill JT, et al. Effects of belimumab, a B lymphocyte stimulator-specific inhibitor, on disease activity across multiple organ domains in patients with systemic lupus erythematosus: combined results from two phase III trials. Ann Rheum Dis 2012;71:1833–8.
32. Tsokos GC, Moutsopoulos HM, Steinberg AD. Muscle involvement in systemic lupus erythematosus. JAMA 1981;246:766–8.
33. Liang Y, Leng RX, Pan HF, et al. Associated variables of myositis in systemic lupus erythematosus: a cross-sectional study. Med Sci Monit 2017;23:2543–9.
34. Tse SM, Mok CC. Time trend and risk factors of avascular bone necrosis in patients with systemic lupus erythematosus. Lupus 2017;26:715–22.
35. Gladman DD, Dhillon N, Su J, et al. Osteonecrosis in SLE: prevalence, patterns, outcomes and predictors. Lupus 2018;27:76–81.

36. Kwon HH, Bang SY, Won S, et al. Synergistic effect of cumulative corticosteroid dose and immunosuppressants on avascular necrosis in patients with systemic lupus erythematosus. Lupus 2018;27:1644–51.
37. Kasturi S, Goodman S. Current perspectives on arthroplasty in systemic lupus erythematosus: rates, outcomes, and adverse events. Curr Rheumatol Rep 2016; 18:59.
38. Bultink IE, Harvey NC, Lalmohamed A, et al. Elevated risk of clinical fractures and associated risk factors in patients with systemic lupus erythematosus versus matched controls: a population-based study in the United Kingdom. Osteoporos Int 2014;25:1275–83.
39. Carli L, Tani C, Spera V, et al. Risk factors for osteoporosis and fragility fractures in patients with systemic lupus erythematosus. Lupus Sci Med 2016;3:e000098.
40. Tedeschi SK, Kim SC, Guan H, et al. Comparative fracture risks among United States Medicaid enrollees with and those without systemic lupus erythematosus. Arthritis Rheumatol 2019;71:1141–6.
41. Aksoy A, Solmaz D, Can G, et al. Increased frequency of hand osteoarthritis in patients with primary Sjögren syndrome compared with systemic lupus erythematosus. J Rheumatol 2016;43:1068–71.
42. Huang FF, Fang R, Nguyen MH, et al. Identifying co-morbid fibromyalgia in patients with systemic lupus erythematosus using the Multi-Dimensional Health Assessment Quectionnaire. Lupus 2020;29:1404–11.
43. Wolfe F, Petri M, Alarcon GS, et al. Fibromyalgia, systemic lupus erythematosus (SLE), and evaluation of SLE activity. J Rheumatol 2009;36:82–8.
44. Clauw DJ. Fibromyalgia: a clinical review. JAMA 2014;311:1547–55.
45. Wolfe F, Clauw DJ, Fitzcharles MA, et al. 2016 revisions to the 2010/2011 fibromyalgia diagnostic criteria. Semin Arthritis Rheum 2016;46:319–29.
46. Wolfe F, Walitt BT, Rasker JJ, et al. The polysymptomatic distress scale is simple, useful, and effective in clinical care and clinical and epidemiology studies. J Rheumatol 2016;43:454.
47. Alunno A, Carubbi F, Stones S, et al. The impact of fibromyalgia in spondyloarthritis: from classification criteria to outcome measures. Front Med 2018;5:290.
48. Cuadrado MJ, Sanna G. Headache and systemic lupus erythematosus. Lupus 2003;12:943–6.
49. Mitsikostas DD, Sfikakis PP, Goadsby PJ. A meta-analysis for headache in systemic lupus erythematosus: the evidence and the myth. Brain 2004;127:1200–9.
50. Lessa B, Santana A, Lima I, et al. Prevalence and classification of headache in patients with systemic lupus erythematosus. Clin Rheumatol 2006;25:850–3.
51. Davey R, Bamford J, Emery P. The ACR classification criteria for headache disorders in SLE fail to classify certain prevalent headache types. Cephalalgia 2008; 28:296–9.
52. The American College of Rheumatology nomenclature and case definitions for neuropsychiatric lupus syndromes. Arthritis Rheum 1999;42:599–608.
53. Gøransson LG, Tjensvoll AB, Herigstad A, et al. Small-diameter nerve fiber neuropathy in systemic lupus erythematosus. Arch Neurol 2006;63:401–4.
54. Bortoluzzi A, Silvagni E, Furini F, et al. Peripheral nervous system involvement in systemic lupus erythematosus: a review of the evidence. Clin Exp Rheumatol 2019;37:146–55.
55. Liu X, Treister R, Lang M, et al. IVIg for apparently autoimmune small-fiber polyneuropathy: first analysis of efficacy and safety. Ther Adv Neurol Disord 2018;11. 1756285617744484.

56. Man BL, Mok CC. Serositis related to systemic lupus erythematosus: prevalence and outcome. Lupus 2005;14:822–6.
57. Dein E, Douglas H, Petri M, et al. Pericarditis in lupus. Cureus 2019;11:e4166.
58. Gladman D, Ginzler E, Goldsmith C, et al. The development and initial validation of the Systemic Lupus International Collaborating Clinics/American College of Rheumatology damage index for systemic lupus erythematosus. Arthritis Rheum 1996;39:363–9.
59. Griffiths B, Mosca M, Gordon C. Assessment of patients with systemic lupus erythematosus and the use of lupus disease activity indices. Best Pract Res Clin Rheumatol 2005;19:685–708.
60. Lam GK, Petri M. Assessment of systemic lupus erythematosus. Clin Exp Rheumatol 2005;23:S120–32.
61. Raison CL, Rutherford RE, Woolwine BJ, et al. A randomized controlled trial of the tumor necrosis factor antagonist infliximab for treatment-resistant depression: the role of baseline inflammatory biomarkers. JAMA Psychiatry 2013;70:31–41.
62. Fleming P, Roubille C, Richer V, et al. Effect of biologics on depressive symptoms in patients with psoriasis: a systematic review. J Eur Acad Dermatol Venereol 2015;29:1063–70.
63. Dantzer R. Cytokine, sickness behavior, and depression. Immunol Allergy Clin North Am 2009;29:247–64.
64. Straub RH, Schradin C. Chronic inflammatory systemic diseases: an evolutionary trade-off between acutely beneficial but chronically harmful programs. Evol Med Public Health 2016;2016:37–51.
65. Straub RH. The brain and immune system prompt energy shortage in chronic inflammation and ageing. Nat Rev Rheumatol 2017;13:743–51.
66. Strand V, Berry P, Lin X, et al. Long-term impact of belimumab on health-related quality of life and fatigue in patients with systemic lupus erythematosus: six years of treatment. Arthritis Care Res 2019;71:829–38.
67. Karol DE, Criscione-Schreiber LG, Lin M, et al. Depressive symptoms and associated factors in systemic lupus erythematosus. Psychosomatics 2013;54:443–50.
68. Eudy AM, Rogers JL, Whitney R, et al. Longitudinal changes in manifestations of SLE (abstract). Arthritis Rheumatol 2019;71(Suppl 10).

Why It Hurts
The Mechanisms of Pain in Rheumatoid Arthritis

Priyanka Iyer, MBBS, MPH[a],*, Yvonne C. Lee, MD, MMSc[b]

KEYWORDS

- Rheumatoid arthritis • Pain mechanisms • Algogens • Central nervous system

KEY POINTS

- Rheumatoid arthritis-related inflammation can reduce the threshold for nociceptors to transmit action potentials, resulting in increased pain sensitivity or hyperalgesia.
- In addition to articular processes, spinal ,and supraspinal processes may play an important role in the modulation of pain in rheumatoid arthritis.
- Immune-mediated processes in rheumatoid arthritis may sensitize the nervous system even before joint inflammation is detected, and this may persist despite the resolution of joint inflammation.
- Quantitative sensory testing and neuroimaging are commonly used methods to study different pain mechanisms in rheumatoid arthritis.

INTRODUCTION

Pain is an important manifestation of inflammation, because inflammatory cytokines and mediators activate and sensitize primary afferent neurons.[1] It should thus not be surprising that pain is nearly a universal feature of rheumatoid arthritis (RA), particularly in those experiencing a flare of the disease. However, ongoing and/or severe inflammation may not suffice to explain pain in some patients with low disease activity who would otherwise be considered to be in remission. It has been noted that up to 40% of patients with RA are regular users of opioid medications,[2,3] with an increase noted in recent years.[2] Although targeted therapies have significantly improved our ability to treat the underlying inflammatory processes and their complications, pain management options have not increased proportionally.

Traditionally, pain in RA was presumed to be primarily driven by peripheral inflammation. One of the first mentions of inflammatory pain was suggested by a 1965 study conducted by Fremont-Smith and Bayles.[4] In this study, the anti-inflammatory effect of acetylsalicylic acid was of greater therapeutic importance than its concurrent analgesic effect in a study of 12 patients with RA who reported improvement in ring size,

[a] Division of Rheumatology, Department of Internal Medicine, University of California Irvine, Irvine, CA, USA; [b] Northwestern University, Chicago, IL, USA
* Corresponding author. Division of Rheumatology, Department of Medicine, 333 City Boulevard, West, Suite 400, Orange, CA 92868.
E-mail address: Priyanka.iyer@mail.harvard.edu

Rheum Dis Clin N Am 47 (2021) 229–244
https://doi.org/10.1016/j.rdc.2020.12.008
0889-857X/21/© 2020 Elsevier Inc. All rights reserved.

rheumatic.theclinics.com

range of motion, grip strength, and finger volume when treated with high-dose acetyl-salicylic acid. However, the recent literature suggests that there is likely a distinct contribution of central pain mechanisms that are in addition to and should be distinguished from that directly arising from peripheral inflammation.[5] When caring for patients with RA, physicians must be familiar with the myriad of contributors to pain. This point is particularly important, because many patients continue to report clinically significant levels of pain despite excellent control of peripheral inflammation.[6]

NOCICEPTION AND TYPES OF PAIN

Pain is a complex and multifaceted experience,[7] composed of both sensory and emotional components.[8] To understand pain, one must first understand nociception, which is the nervous system's process of encoding noxious stimuli owing to impending or actual tissue damage.[1] Nociception contributes to the pain experience but is not equivalent to pain,[7] which is a highly individualized experience that is impacted by multiple factors, including sleep, psychosocial distress, and past circumstances.[2]

Pain can be subdivided into 3 broad categories that may be particularly applicable for those with rheumatic diseases.[9] Nociceptive pain arises from actual or threatened damage to non-neural tissue and occurs as a result of the activation of nociceptors. In contrast, neuropathic pain is caused by a lesion or disease of the somatosensory nervous system. More recently, a new descriptor of pain, termed nociplastic pain, was added to the taxonomy. Nociplastic pain is defined as pain that arises from altered nociception despite there being no clear evidence of actual or threatened tissue damage or a lesion of the somatosensory system.[10] Nociplastic pain may be relevant to certain patients seen in the rheumatology clinic, particularly those with nonspecific back pain, nonspecific peripheral joint pain, and fibromyalgia.[9] Some pain specialists also use the term mixed pain to define pain with an overlap of nociceptive and neuropathic symptoms.[11]

In this article, we discuss the current understanding of mechanisms that contribute to nociception and the experience of pain in RA.

PERIPHERAL MECHANISMS OF PAIN: INFLAMMATORY CYTOKINES AND MORE

Noxious stimuli are transmitted by rapidly conducting Aδ and slow conducting C fibers that innervate the joint and increase their firing rate in response to activation at nerve terminals. These fibers transmit impulses through the peripheral nerve up through the dorsal root and centrally into the dorsal horn of the spinal cord. The Aδ fibers relay first or fast pain and terminate in the superficial dorsal horn, whereas the C fibers relay second or slow pain and terminate predominantly in deeper structures in the spinal cord.

Inflammatory events in RA activate cells of both the adaptive and innate immune systems, producing a cascade of inflammatory mediators and attracting neutrophils, T cells, and B cells to the synovium, resulting in synovitis. The inflamed synovium generates multiple algogens, including bioactive lipids, kinins, cytokines (eg, tumor necrosis factor [TNF]-α, IL-1, and IL-6), neuropeptides (eg, calcitonin gene-related peptide), and neurotrophins (eg, nerve growth factor).[12-15] These signaling molecules can activate and sensitize nociceptors in the synovium, joint capsule, ligaments, subchondral bone, tendon sheaths, and muscles. Nerve growth factor, in particular, has received significant recent attention, because it promotes the proliferation of terminal nerves, upregulates the release of substance P, and contributes to the degranulation of mast cells leading to the release of histamine that activates nociceptor nerve terminals.[13]

In response to noxious inflammatory stimuli, ligand-gated and voltage-gated ion channels (eg, transient receptor potential V1 and Nav 1.7) are activated on the nociceptor nerve terminals.[16,17] Cytokines such as IL-1β, IL-6, TNF-α, and IL-17 act via signaling mechanisms to potentiate transient receptor potential and Nav channel activation, leading to the rapid sensitization of nociceptor neurons.[17] Neutrophils release neutrophil elastase, which cleaves proteinase-activated receptor 2, a G-protein–coupled receptor expressed on joint sensory nerves.[18] The activation of proteinase-activated receptor 2 results in the generation of joint pain and peripheral sensitization in rats and mice.[18–21] Nociceptors also actively release neuropeptides that modulate the activity of innate and adaptive immune cells,[22] suggesting bidirectional interactions between nociceptors and immune cells.[17] As a result of inflammation in RA, the threshold for nociceptor neurons to fire action potentials is decreased, leading to increased pain sensitivity or hyperalgesia.[22]

Animal models indicate that mechanical hypersensitivity often precedes and outlasts joint inflammation, suggesting the presence of additional noninflammatory etiologies for pain.[23] In a collagen antibody-induced arthritis model, mice developed transient joint inflammation, but pain-like behavior was observed before and outlasted the visual signs of arthritis. This finding may be the result of a greater concentration of nerve fibers in the synovium and the aberrant firing of afferent nerves. In a recent mouse study with the K/BxN model, researchers identified an increased density of nerve fibers in the synovium of arthritic ankles and also discovered that nerve fibers have a sprouted disorganized appearance that may lead to spontaneous discharges.[24] These observations suggest a potential role for sensory and sympathetic nerve fiber remodeling in the generation and maintenance of arthritic pain. A recent mouse K/BxN serum transfer model study also suggested that a decrease in the expression of proresolving lipid mediators may contribute to allodynia that persists after the resolution of joint swelling.[25]

CENTRAL MECHANISMS OF PAIN

Central sensitization was first described by Clifford Woolf in 1983 when he observed that enhanced, postinjury responses to sural nerve stimulation remained after blocking peripheral sensation with local anesthesia, indicating a role for then central nervous system (CNS) modulation of pain.[26] Since then, multiple mechanisms of central sensitization have been elucidated, which involve both spinal and supraspinal pathways. Although it is likely that these mechanisms play a role in the development and maintenance of chronic pain in RA, it is important to note that the majority of data discussed in this section are not specific to RA or other systemic inflammatory conditions.

Spinal modulation of pain perception occurs in the dorsal horn of the spinal cord, where primary nociceptive afferents terminate, and the incoming signals are transmitted to projection neurons for relay to the brain. At the dorsal horn, central sensitization can occur via multiple pathways, including (1) an increase in presynaptic excitatory neurotransmitter (eg, glutamate, substance P) release, (2) enhancement of the postsynaptic response (eg, at the N-methyl-D-aspartate receptor and/or G-protein–coupled receptors), (3) dampening of inhibitory neurotransmitters (eg, gamma aminobutyric acid and/or glycine), and (4) enhancement of membrane excitability (such that stimuli that would normally be subthreshold induce the propagation of action potentials).[14,27]

In addition, recent studies have implicated spinal microglia and astrocytes as important contributors to the CNS modulation of pain.[28] Spinal microglia express receptors for adenosine triphosphate and CX3CL1. Activation of these receptors upregulates the production of TNF-α, IL-1β, IL-18, brain-derived growth factor, and cyclo-oxygenase.[29,30] In a collagen-induced rat arthritis model of inflammatory arthritis, reactive spinal microgliosis occurred with a similar time course as the development of mechanical hypersensitivity, at least 1 week before the onset of joint swelling and other clinical signs of arthritis.[31] Concurrent with the development of spinal microgliosis and mechanical hypersensitivity, increases in IL-1β levels were also observed in the cerebrospinal fluid. Intriguingly, there is also clinical evidence that proinflammatory cytokines, including IL-1β, are increased in the cerebrospinal fluid of patients with RA.[32,33]

Studies have also shown that spinal astrocytes are capable of synthesizing proinflammatory cytokines (eg, IL-1β), growth factors (eg, fibroblast growth factor 2), proteases (eg, matrix metalloproteinase 2), and chemokines (CCL2, CCL7, and CXCL1) that are important for the maintenance of chronic pain.[34–39] However, in the same rat model that showed reactive microgliosis in the early stages of collagen-induced arthritis, no increases in activated astrocytes were noted.[31] Additional studies are needed to clarify the role of astrocytes in the CNS modulation of pain in the setting of inflammatory arthritis.

From the dorsal horn, nociceptive signals are carried along the ascending pain pathways to the brain stem, hypothalamus, thalamus, and cerebral cortex by second-order dorsal neurons.[40] The spinothalamic tract plays an important role in transmitting information to the somatosensory cortex, thus providing information on the intensity and the location of the noxious stimulus. Other projection neurons engage the cingulate and insular cortices via the connections in the parabrachial nucleus and the amygdala, hence contributing to the pain experience.[41]

Descending pathways arise from areas in the brain located in the cortex (mainly the periaqueductal gray), hypothalamus, and brain stem (rostral ventromedial medulla), and modulate sensory input from the primary afferent fibers and projection neurons in the dorsal horn of the spinal cord.[42] Several descending pathways are activated in response to noxious stimuli and can cause a widespread decrease in pain sensitivity after exposure to acutely painful stimuli. These inhibitory pathways may be impaired in subgroups of patients with systemic inflammatory conditions like RA and might additionally contribute to the development of chronic pain.[43]

ASSESSING PAIN IN RHEUMATOID ARTHRITIS

The assessment of patients with pain in RA may use the following methods: patient-reported measures, quantitative sensory testing (QST), and functional neuroimaging (functional MRI [fMRI] and PET).

Measures Based on Patient Report

The most commonly used measure to assess pain is a rating of pain intensity, as assessed by a visual analog scale or numeric rating scale.[44] Other frequently used measures of pain assessment include validated assessments of pain and pain-related constructs using the Patient-Reported Outcomes Measurement Information System.[45,46] These instruments include item banks to assess pain interference, pain behavior, and pain quality.[47–49] Other legacy instruments commonly used to assess pain include the Brief Pain Inventory,[50,51] the McGill Pain Questionnaire,[52,53] and the Short Form-36 Bodily Pain Scale.[54]

In addition, measures to assess noninflammatory pain and, more specifically, the concepts of fibromyalgianess, central sensitization, and neuropathic pain, have been developed. To assess noninflammatory pain, McWilliams and colleagues[55] developed a measure that reflects the proportion of the Disease Activity Score in 28 joints (DAS28) attributable to patient-reported components (DAS28-P). The DAS28-P is calculated by dividing the portion of the DAS28 contributed by the tender joint count and the patient global assessment by the total DAS28 score. McWilliams and colleagues found that patients with high DAS28-P scores had a lesser likelihood of pain improvement. Based on this observation, the authors suggested that the DAS28-P may represent pain sensitization owing to central causes, such as fibromyalgia, rather than inflammation itself. A separate study found that the DAS28-P had very good discriminatory power for identifying patients with RA and secondary fibromyalgia compared with those with RA alone.[56]

To diagnose fibromyalgia, Wolfe and colleagues[57,58] developed the American College of Rheumatology 2010/2011 Preliminary Diagnostic Criteria for Fibromyalgia, which is composed of the Widespread Pain Index and the Symptom Severity Score. The Fibromyalgia Survey Questionnaire, which consists of the Widespread Pain Index and Symptom Severity Score, was subsequently evaluated as a measure of fibromyalgia severity.[59] Although not formally validated in patients with RA, this measure was developed in a population that included patients with RA, and several studies have shown that it is associated with poor outcomes, including disability, quality of life, and disease activity measures among patients with RA.[60–62] It should be noted that the Fibromyalgia Survey Questionnaire was originally termed the Polysymptomatic Distress Scale. Thus, several publications refer to it under the previous name.

The Central Sensitization Inventory (CSI) is another questionnaire-based method of assessing centralized pain.[63] Similar to the Fibromyalgia Survey Questionnaire, the CSI asks about symptoms associated with central sensitization (eg, headaches, feeling unrefreshed, depression), as well as pain in multiple locations (eg, pain all over the body, pain in the jaw, and pain in the pelvic area). Construct validity was established by comparing scores in patients with fibromyalgia, chronic widespread pain without fibromyalgia, work-related regional chronic low back pain, and a normative control group.[63] Compared with the Fibromyalgia Survey Questionnaire, the CSI has not been used as frequently in rheumatic disease populations. A study of 193 patients with 1 of 4 rheumatic conditions (RA, spondyloarthropathy, osteoarthritis, or fibromyalgia) reported that central sensitization, defined by the CSI, was identified in 41% of patients with RA, 45% of patients with spondyloarthropathy, 62% of patients with osteoarthritis, and 94% of patients with fibromyalgia.[64] However, the authors did not specify the thresholds used to define central sensitization in this study.

The painDETECT questionnaire has also been used to characterize pain in patients with RA. This questionnaire was originally developed to assess neuropathic pain in patients with back pain,[65] but has been applied in studies of multiple other conditions, including RA. A Rasch analysis of 900 questionnaires indicated acceptable psychometric properties among patients with RA, spondyloarthropathy, and psoriatic arthritis.[66] In several studies of patients with RA, the prevalence of neuropathic pain, defined by a painDETECT score of 19 or higher, ranging from 3% to 20%, with another 11% to 28% with painDETECT scores from 13 to 18.[67–69] In cross-sectional studies, painDETECT scores were associated with self-reported pain intensity and composite disease activity measures, but not with objective measures of inflammation, such as swollen joint count and C-reactive protein.[68,70] As a result, it was suggested that high painDETECT scores may indicate a noninflammatory or non-nociceptive mechanism. Longitudinal studies, however, have been conflicting. Two studies (one in early RA and one in established RA) reported that high painDETECT scores were associated with a lower likelihood of achieving disease remission.[71,72] In contrast, a study of 102 patients with RA starting a disease-modifying antirheumatic drug (DMARD) did not show any association between high painDETECT scores and change in disease activity (measured by the DAS28), change in an MRI-based synovitis score, or change in pain intensity measured by visual analog scale.[67] However, the sample size of patients with high painDETECT scores was small (n = 17) and may have limited the ability to detect meaningful differences in outcomes.[67]

Although helpful in characterizing pain and pain-related constructs, these questionnaires have several limitations. First, although they can assess the symptoms of clinical conditions associated with central sensitization (eg, fibromyalgia), they ultimately do not provide information on the mechanisms underlying these symptoms. Few studies have examined the correlations between these measures and other assessments of central sensitization (eg, the QST).[73,74] Besides, most of these questionnaires were developed in noninflammatory pain conditions or heterogeneous populations that included both inflammatory and noninflammatory pain conditions. Thus, the applicability of these measures to patients with RA, particularly those with active inflammatory joint disease is unclear.

Quantitative Sensory Testing

The QST is a set of semiquantitative, noninvasive methods for the assessment of nervous system sensitization to nociceptive signaling by assessing response to quantifiable noxious stimuli.[75] Pressure pain thresholds (PPTs), temporal summation (TS), and conditioned pain modulation (CPM) are the most widely used QST paradigms.

Pain threshold

The point at which a sensation first becomes painful is called the pain threshold. Higher pain thresholds reflect lower pain sensitivity. Several types of stimuli can be used to assess pain thresholds, including pressure, heat, cold, and vibration.

One of the most commonly modalities used stimuli to assess pain thresholds in RA is pressure, because it is thought to be most reflective of arthritis pain. An algometer probe is pressed against a predefined area of skin, and a series of ascending stimulus intensities are applied until pain is reported and the pressure pain-detection threshold (PPT) is identified. Low PPTs at joint sites are thought to indicate increased pain sensitivity as a result of local inflammation, whereas low PPTs at nonjoint sites are considered indicative of central sensitization.[76]

Studies assessing PPTs have provided evidence supporting the existence of peripheral sensitization at joint sites among patients with RA.[43,77,78] We and others have demonstrated that, compared with pain-free controls, patients with RA report lower PPTs at joint sites. Among patients with RA, PPTs at joint sites are consistently associated with tender joint count.[79,80] In a study of 59 patients with established RA, we also observed an association between PPT at the wrist and serum C-reactive protein levels, consistent with peripheral sensitization.[81] In contrast, we did not observe an association between PPTs at joint sites and swollen joint count in a larger study of 139 patients with active RA.[80] Similarly, Joharatnam and colleagues[79] did not observe an association between PPT at the knee and either swollen joint count or the erythrocyte sedimentation rate. The reason for this discrepancy is not clear. In these studies, PPTs were assessed at specific joint sites, irrespective of actual joint inflammation. Thus, it is possible that the joints assessed by QST were not inflamed and others were inflamed. Additional studies are needed to assess the association between peripheral inflammation and PPTs in patients with RA.

Studies assessing PPTs also suggest that patients with RA have abnormalities consistent with central sensitization.[43,82,83] The primary evidence for central sensitization is the observation that PPTs at nonjoint sites are diffusely lower among patients with RA compared with healthy controls. The clinical relevance of these data is underscored by the observation that low extra-articular PPTs are associated with overall pain intensity, even after adjustment for C-reactive protein level and swollen joint count.[84] Low extra-articular PPTs are also associated with pain-related measures of RA disease activity (eg, a high tender joint count, a high patient global assessment, and a high Crohn's Disease Activity Index), but not objective measures of inflammation (eg, swollen joint count).[80] These studies point toward a role for pain centralization as a contributor to the pain experience in patients with RA. Given the assumption that pain in RA is related to inflammation, central sensitization also seems to contribute to higher composite measures of disease activity, despite the lack of association between extra-articular PPTs and objective measures of inflammation.

Temporal summation

TS occurs as a result of the summation of C fiber responses with brief intervals between stimuli. When the initial postsynaptic potential does not fully resolve before the onset of the next stimulus, there is a progressive increase in the perception of pain, even though subsequent stimuli are of the same magnitude as the first. This process mimics the initial wind-up process of dorsal horn neurons to peripheral stimulation and is an important mechanism of central sensitization.[85]

Two small studies have reported that patients with RA experience higher TS of pain than healthy controls. In a study comparing TS in 11 patients with RA, 10 patients with fibromyalgia, and 20 healthy, pain-free participants, Hermans and colleagues[86] reported that the TS was higher among the subgroups with RA and fibromyalgia, compared with healthy, pain-free participants. Additionally, Vladimirova and colleagues[87] noted a greater TS in 38 patients with RA with active disease compared with 38 healthy female control participants. In a study of 263 patients with RA, our research group reported a significant association between TS and patient-reported pain, with higher pain intensity in the most centrally dysregulated TS group compared with the least dysregulated group.[84] Greater central pain dysregulation was also significantly associated with more pain interference in unadjusted analyses, which was attenuated in the adjusted analysis. An analysis of a subset of these patients also revealed that high TS was associated with high tender joint counts, a high patient global assessment, a high evaluator global assessment, and a higher Crohn's Disease Activity Index.[80] Taken together, these studies suggest that an enhanced TS of pain may be a key pathway underlying the central pain dysregulation in RA.

Interestingly, however, TS has not been associated with poor treatment response in RA. Our research group did not see a statistically significant association between TS and European League Against Rheumatism response in a study of 182 patients.[88] Similarly, Christensen and colleagues[89] did not find a statistically significant association between TS and change in DAS28 at 4 months after DMARD initiation. Thus, although patients with RA seem to have an enhanced TS of pain, this mechanism does not seem to impact pain longitudinally. It is possible that the resolution of inflammation with DMARD treatment also leads to improvements in the TS. Additional studies are underway to explore this possibility.

Conditioned modulation

CPM refers to the concept that "pain inhibits pain."[90] Noxious input from peripheral C-fibers activates inhibitory pathways in the brain and spinal cord to diffusely inhibit incoming noxious stimuli.[91,92] In the laboratory, the initial noxious stimulus (test stimulus) is measured before and after the application of a second stimulus (conditioning stimulus), which activates the inhibitory pathways. In healthy individuals with properly functioning descending inhibitory pain pathways, the postconditioning test stimulus is perceived as less painful than the preconditioning test stimulus because the conditioning stimulus activates the descending inhibitory pathways leading to a decrease in pain sensitivity. In individuals with chronic pain conditions, the descending inhibitory pain pathways may not function appropriately.[93] As a result, the decrease in pain sensitivity after exposure to the conditioning stimulus may be diminished.

Data regarding CPM in patients with RA have been conflicting. Hermans and colleagues[86] reported no difference in CPM between patients with RA (n = 11) compared with healthy controls (n = 20). However, in a study of 58 female patients with RA and 54 age-matched, female healthy controls, our research group reported that patients with RA experienced impaired CPM (median, 0.5 kg/cm^2) compared with healthy controls (median, 1.5 kg/cm^2).[43] Using mediation analyses, the same authors noted that low CPM levels in patients with RA may be attributed in part to sleep disturbances. This study was cross-sectional, so no causal inferences could be made.

Among patients with RA, impaired CPM has been associated with higher tender joint counts,[80] but not overall pain intensity.[84] The reason for this discrepancy is not clear, but may be related to differences in the measures of pain, with the tender joint count being a disease-specific measure and overall pain intensity reflecting multiple potential causes of bodily pain. Of note, our research group recently demonstrated that patients with RA with a low CPM were significantly less likely to have a good response to DMARD treatment.[88] These results suggest that inefficient CNS pain inhibition may contribute to a heightened assessment of disease activity, possibly by increasing subjective, disease-related, pain measures, such as the tender joint count.

Although it is still not clear how to improve CPM among patients with RA, a small study suggested that exercise does not improve CPM.[94] The same study also evaluated the effects of acetaminophen on CPM, but the results were inconsistent.[95] Additional studies are needed to identify efficacious interventions for improving CPM in patients with RA.

Neuroimaging Evidence

Recent advances in neuroimaging have identified differences in the structure and function of the brain in patients with RA compared with healthy, pain-free controls.[96,97] Wartolowska and colleagues[98] conducted an MRI study to investigate the brain correlates of pain in an RA population compared with healthy controls. They used a technique called voxel-based morphometry, which revealed larger gray matter volume in the caudate nucleus, putamen, and nucleus accumbens of patients with RA compared with controls. These structures are important in the cognitive, affective, and sensory discriminative processing of pain. These findings could represent chronic changes in the brain structures in response to long-term exposure to pain. Alternatively, these differences could also be attributed to other factors that differ between patients and controls (eg, inflammation, medications, and physical activity levels).

In addition, a growing body of evidence suggests that patients with RA may exhibit functional changes in the brain in response to pain.[99] Our research group used arterial spin labeling (ASL) to identify changes in the regional cerebral blood flow (rCBF) associated with pain provocations in patients with RA and pain-free control participants.[100] ASL is a noninvasive fMRI technique that enables quantifiable measurement of rCBF as a proxy for neural activation.[101] Joint pain was exacerbated by inflating a pressure cuff around the metacarpophalangeal joints for 6 minutes. In response to this stimulus, rCBF in the medial frontal cortex and the dorsolateral prefrontal cortex (dlPFC) increased among patients with RA. In contrast, no changes in the rCBF were noted in pain-free controls. These results suggest that the medial frontal cortex and the dlPFC may be areas of particular relevance to disease-related pain in RA.

Of note, the dlPFC was also highlighted as a region involved in RA-related pain in a recent study of 31 patients with RA and 23 controls.[102] In this study, participants underwent fMRI while being exposed to a series of painful and nonpainful pressure stimuli for 2.5 seconds each. Interestingly, this study showed deactivation (as opposed to activation) of the dlPFC in response to painful pressure. The authors postulated that the difference in results between this study and the ASL study mentioned elsewhere in this article may have been due to the duration of the noxious stimuli. When patients with RA are exposed to longer durations of noxious stimuli (as in the ASL study), the inhibition of pain through the dlPFC may be activated, whereas when participants are exposed to short pulses of noxious stimuli, the tonic inhibition of pain may be temporarily inactivated. Thus, patients may still feel acute increases in pain owing to acute noxious insults, thereby prompting the removal of the inflamed joint from potentially tissue-damaging situations, while simultaneously allowing the patient to acclimate to long-standing noxious stimuli. Additional studies are needed to clarify the role of the dlPFC in responding to noxious pain stimuli in patients with RA.

In addition to the differences in the rCBF and the neural activity in specific brain regions, recent studies suggest that patients with RA may exhibit differences in the way brain regions are connected functionally. Functional brain connectivity refers to the synchronization of neural activity displayed by 2 or more brain regions. It is assumed that this synchronization reflects communication between the brain regions.

Among patients with RA, systemic inflammation may be associated with changes in functional connectivity between the default mode network and other brain regions associated with pain. The default mode network is a group of interconnected brain regions that includes the medial prefrontal cortex, posterior cingulate cortex, precuneus, inferior parietal lobule, hippocampal formation, and lateral temporal cortex.[103] Functional connectivity between the default mode network and the insula has previously been identified as a neurobiological feature of primary fibromyalgia.[104–106] In a cross-sectional analysis of 54 patients with RA, Schrepf and colleagues[99] observed that erythrocyte sedimentation rate levels were positively correlated with functional connections between the inferior parietal lobule, medial prefrontal cortex, and several brain networks. Using data from the same population, Kaplan and colleagues[107] observed significant associations between erythrocyte sedimentation rate levels and the left inferior parietal lobule–insula functional connectivity, the left inferior parietal lobule–dorsal anterior cingulate functional connectivity, and the left inferior parietal lobule–medial prefrontal cortex functional connectivity among patients with RA with fibromyalgia, but not in patients with RA without fibromyalgia. A third report, also using data from the same 54 patients with RA, reported associations between functional connectivity between the default mode network and insula and the symptoms of fibromyalgia.[108] Taken together, these studies suggest that systemic inflammation may lead to changes in brain functional connectivity, which are associated with the development of a centrally sensitized state, that is, secondary fibromyalgia, among patients with RA. However, it should be noted that these analyses were all cross-sectional, and the study population consisted of patients with RA with an average disease duration of 11.5 years. Future studies involving longitudinal analyses in patients with a recent onset of the disease are needed to clarify the potential role of systemic inflammation in precipitating functional changes related to the acute to chronic pain transition in patients with RA.

In addition to understanding the neurobiological underpinnings of chronic pain in RA, fMRI studies have also provided evidence for how TNF-α inhibition can alleviate pain symptoms in patients with RA, even before changes in inflammation are observed. Rech and colleagues[109] conducted evoked pain fMRI in 10 patients with

RA before and after anti-TNF therapy with certolizumab and observed the differences in brain activation between responders and nonresponders. Compared with nonresponders, responders showed a significantly higher baseline activation in the thalamic, limbic, and associative areas of the brain. Brain activity in these areas decreased within 3 days after exposure to a TNF inhibitor in the responders, preceding clinical responses, and those noted on the anatomic hand MRI. This work again implies the possible existence of different neural signatures for different types of pain, because responders are more likely than nonresponders to have pain originating from inflammation. The lack of a control group and a small sample size are some of the limitations of these studies. Further studies are needed before conclusions can be made regarding the role of TNF-α inhibitors on the CNS regulation of pain.

FUTURE AREAS OF RESEARCH

Although the underlying mechanisms for pain in RA are beginning to be elucidated, the effect of treatment with DMARDs on the different types of pain in RA, the peripheral and central components of pain, and the role of centrally active antihyperalgesics on pain still needs to be identified. This work will be of great significance in the development of new analgesic therapeutics for RA.

CLINICS CARE POINTS

- In addition to peripheral joint inflammation, health care providers should consider other potential causes of pain, such as abnormalities in the CNS regulation of pain.
- Despite the perception of patients with RA being very stoic and resistant to pain, patients with RA are more sensitive to pain than healthy, pain-free individuals.
- To assess noninflammatory pain in RA in the clinic, health care providers could consider using measures based on patient-reported pain and symptoms, such as the DAS28-P, Fibromyalgia Survey Questionnaire, Central Sensitization Index, or painDETECT.
- If patients present with widespread pain but minimal joint inflammation, health care providers should consider treatments targeted at centralized pain mechanisms rather than aggressively increasing immunosuppressive therapies.

DISCLOSURE

P. Iyer: Have nothing to disclose. Y.C. Lee: Research support from Pfizer; consulting for Highland Instruments; stock in Cigna-Express Scripts; unpaid consulting for Sanofi and Eli Lilly.

REFERENCES

1. Zhang JM. An J. Cytokines, inflammation, and pain. Int Anesthesiol Clin 2007; 45(2):27–37.
2. Zamora-Legoff JA, Achenbach SJ, Crowson CS, et al. Opioid use in patients with rheumatoid arthritis 2005-2014: a population-based comparative study. Clin Rheumatol 2016;35(5):1137–44.
3. Curtis JR, Xie F, Smith C, et al. Changing trends in opioid use among patients with rheumatoid arthritis in the United States. Arthritis Rheumatol 2017;69(9): 1733–40.

4. Fremont-Smith K, Bayles TB. Salicylate therapy in rheumatoid arthritis. JAMA 1965;192:1133–6.
5. Zhang A, Lee YC. Mechanisms for joint pain in rheumatoid arthritis (RA): from cytokines to central sensitization. Curr Osteoporos Rep 2018;16(5):603–10.
6. Taylor P, Manger B, Alvaro-Gracia J, et al. Patient perceptions concerning pain management in the treatment of rheumatoid arthritis. J Int Med Res 2010;38(4):1213–24.
7. Roditi D, Robinson ME. The role of psychological interventions in the management of patients with chronic pain. Psychol Res Behav Manag 2011;4:41–9.
8. Merskey HBN, editor. Classification of chronic pain. 2nd edition. Seattle, WA: IASP Press; 1994. p. 209–14. Task Force on Taxonomy of the IASP Part III: pain terms, a current list with definitions and notes on usage.
9. Trouvin AP, Perrot S. New concepts of pain. Best Pract Res Clin Rheumatol 2019;33(3):101415.
10. Nociplastic pain. Available at: https://www.iasp-pain.org/Education/Content.aspx?ItemNumber=1698#Nociplasticpain. Accessed November 1, 2020.
11. Freynhagen R, Parada HA, Calderon-Ospina CA, et al. Current understanding of the mixed pain concept: a brief narrative review. Curr Med Res Opin 2019;35(6):1011–8.
12. Konttinen YT, Tiainen VM, Gomez-Barrena E, et al. Innervation of the joint and role of neuropeptides. Ann N Y Acad Sci 2006;1069:149–54.
13. Raychaudhuri SP, Raychaudhuri SK, Atkuri KR, ot al. Nerve growth factor: a key local regulator in the pathogenesis of inflammatory arthritis. Arthritis Rheum 2011;63(11):3243–52.
14. Schaible HG, Ebersberger A, Von Banchet GS. Mechanisms of pain in arthritis. Ann N Y Acad Sci 2002;966:343–54.
15. Schaible HG, von Banchet GS, Boettger MK, et al. The role of proinflammatory cytokines in the generation and maintenance of joint pain. Ann N Y Acad Sci 2010;1193:60–9.
16. Basbaum AI, Bautista DM, Scherrer G, et al. Cellular and molecular mechanisms of pain. Cell 2009;139(2):267–84.
17. Chiu IM, von Hehn CA, Woolf CJ. Neurogenic inflammation and the peripheral nervous system in host defense and immunopathology. Nat Neurosci 2012;15(8):1063–7.
18. Steinhoff M, Vergnolle N, Young SH, et al. Agonists of proteinase-activated receptor 2 induce inflammation by a neurogenic mechanism. Nat Med 2000;6(2):151–8.
19. Helyes Z, Sandor K, Borbely E, et al. Involvement of transient receptor potential vanilloid 1 receptors in protease-activated receptor-2-induced joint inflammation and nociception. Eur J Pain 2010;14(4):351–8.
20. Russell FA, McDougall JJ. Proteinase activated receptor (PAR) involvement in mediating arthritis pain and inflammation. Inflamm Res 2009;58(3):119–26.
21. Russell FA, Veldhoen VE, Tchitchkan D, et al. Proteinase-activated receptor-4 (PAR4) activation leads to sensitization of rat joint primary afferents via a bradykinin B2 receptor-dependent mechanism. J Neurophysiol 2010;103(1):155–63.
22. Pinho-Ribeiro FA, Verri WA Jr, Chiu IM. Nociceptor Sensory Neuron-Immune Interactions in Pain and Inflammation. Trends Immunol 2017;38(1):5–19.
23. Bas DB, Su J, Sandor K, et al. Collagen antibody-induced arthritis evokes persistent pain with spinal glial involvement and transient prostaglandin dependency. Arthritis Rheum 2012;64(12):3886–96.

24. Goncalves Dos Santos G, Jimenez-Andrade JM, Woller SA, et al. The neuropathic phenotype of the K/BxN transgenic mouse with spontaneous arthritis: pain, nerve sprouting and joint remodeling. Sci Rep 2020;10(1):15596.

25. Allen BL, Montague-Cardoso K, Simeoli R, et al. Imbalance of pro-resolving lipid mediators in persistent allodynia dissociated from signs of clinical arthritis. Pain 2020;161(9):2155–66.

26. Woolf CJ. Evidence for a central component of post-injury pain hypersensitivity. Nature 1983;306(5944):686–8.

27. Woolf CJ. Central sensitization: implications for the diagnosis and treatment of pain. Pain 2011;152(3 Suppl):S2–15.

28. Milligan ED, Watkins LR. Pathological and protective roles of glia in chronic pain. Nat Rev Neurosci 2009;10(1):23–36.

29. Coull JA, Beggs S, Boudreau D, et al. BDNF from microglia causes the shift in neuronal anion gradient underlying neuropathic pain. Nature 2005;438(7070): 1017–21.

30. Ji RR, Chamessian A, Zhang YQ. Pain regulation by non-neuronal cells and inflammation. Science 2016;354(6312):572–7.

31. Nieto FR, Clark AK, Grist J, et al. Neuron-immune mechanisms contribute to pain in early stages of arthritis. J Neuroinflammation 2016;13(1):96.

32. Lampa J, Westman M, Kadetoff D, et al. Peripheral inflammatory disease associated with centrally activated IL-1 system in humans and mice. Proc Natl Acad Sci U S A 2012;109(31):12728–33.

33. Kosek E, Altawil R, Kadetoff D, et al. Evidence of different mediators of central inflammation in dysfunctional and inflammatory pain- interleukin-8 in fibromyalgia and interleukin-1 beta in rheumatoid arthritis. J Neuroimmunol 2015;280: 49–55.

34. Gao YJ, Ji RR. Targeting astrocyte signaling for chronic pain. Neurotherapeutics 2010;7(4):482–93.

35. Gao YJ, Zhang L, Samad OA, et al. JNK-induced MCP-1 production in spinal cord astrocytes contributes to central sensitization and neuropathic pain. J Neurosci 2009;29(13):4096–108.

36. Guo W, Wang H, Watanabe M, et al. Glial-cytokine-neuronal interactions underlying the mechanisms of persistent pain. J Neurosci 2007;27(22):6006–18.

37. Imai S, Ikegami D, Yamashita A, et al. Epigenetic transcriptional activation of monocyte chemotactic protein 3 contributes to long-lasting neuropathic pain. Brain 2013;136(Pt 3):828–43.

38. Kawasaki Y, Xu ZZ, Wang X, et al. Distinct roles of matrix metalloproteases in the early- and late-phase development of neuropathic pain. Nat Med 2008;14(3): 331–6.

39. Deng Y, Lu J, Li W, et al. Reciprocal inhibition of YAP/TAZ and NF-kappaB regulates osteoarthritic cartilage degradation. Nat Commun 2018;9(1):4564.

40. Hunter DJ, McDougall JJ, Keefe FJ. The symptoms of osteoarthritis and the genesis of pain. Rheum Dis Clin North Am 2008;34(3):623–43.

41. Bushnell MC, Ceko M, Low LA. Cognitive and emotional control of pain and its disruption in chronic pain. Nat Rev Neurosci 2013;14(7):502–11.

42. Ossipov MH, Dussor GO, Porreca F. Central modulation of pain. J Clin Invest 2010;120(11):3779–87.

43. Lee YC, Lu B, Edwards RR, et al. The role of sleep problems in central pain processing in rheumatoid arthritis. Arthritis Rheum 2013;65(1):59–68.

44. Hawker GA, Mian S, Kendzerska T, et al. Measures of adult pain: Visual Analog Scale for Pain (VAS Pain), Numeric Rating Scale for Pain (NRS Pain), McGill Pain

Questionnaire (MPQ), Short-Form McGill Pain Questionnaire (SF-MPQ), Chronic Pain Grade Scale (CPGS), Short Form-36 Bodily Pain Scale (SF-36 BPS), and Measure of Intermittent and Constant Osteoarthritis Pain (ICOAP). Arthritis Care Res (Hoboken) 2011;63(Suppl 11):S240–52.

45. Crins MHP, Terwee CB, Westhovens R, et al. First Validation of the Full PROMIS pain interference and pain behavior item banks in patients with rheumatoid arthritis. Arthritis Care Res (Hoboken) 2020;72(11):1550–9.

46. Bykerk VP. Patient-reported outcomes measurement information system versus legacy instruments: are they ready for prime time? Rheum Dis Clin North Am 2019;45(2):211–29.

47. Amtmann D, Cook KF, Jensen MP, et al. Development of a PROMIS item bank to measure pain interference. Pain 2010;150(1):173–82.

48. Revicki DA, Chen WH, Harnam N, et al. Development and psychometric analysis of the PROMIS pain behavior item bank. Pain 2009;146(1–2):158–69.

49. Revicki DA, Cook KF, Amtmann D, et al. Exploratory and confirmatory factor analysis of the PROMIS pain quality item bank. Qual Life Res 2014;23(1): 245–55.

50. Tan G, Jensen MP, Thornby JI, et al. Validation of the Brief Pain Inventory for chronic nonmalignant pain. J Pain 2004;5(2):133–7.

51. Cleeland CS, Ryan KM. Pain assessment: global use of the Brief Pain Inventory. Ann Acad Med Singap 1994;23(2):129–38.

52. Burckhardt CS. The use of the McGill Pain Questionnaire in assessing arthritis pain. Pain 1984;19(3):305–14.

53. Melzack R. The short-form McGill Pain Questionnaire. Pain 1987;30(2):191–7.

54. McHorney CA, Ware JE Jr, Raczek AE. The MOS 36-Item Short-Form Health Survey (SF-36): II. Psychometric and clinical tests of validity in measuring physical and mental health constructs. Med Care 1993;31(3):247–63.

55. McWilliams DF, Zhang W, Mansell JS, et al. Predictors of change in bodily pain in early rheumatoid arthritis: an inception cohort study. Arthritis Care Res (Hoboken) 2012;64(10):1505–13.

56. Salaffi F, Di Carlo M, Carotti M, et al. The subjective components of the Disease Activity Score 28-joints (DAS28) in rheumatoid arthritis patients and coexisting fibromyalgia. Rheumatol Int 2018;38(10):1911–8.

57. Wolfe F, Clauw DJ, Fitzcharles MA, et al. The American College of Rheumatology preliminary diagnostic criteria for fibromyalgia and measurement of symptom severity. Arthritis Care Res (Hoboken) 2010;62(5):600–10.

58. Wolfe F, Clauw DJ, Fitzcharles MA, et al. Fibromyalgia criteria and severity scales for clinical and epidemiological studies: a modification of the ACR Preliminary Diagnostic Criteria for Fibromyalgia. J Rheumatol 2011;38(6):1113–22.

59. Hauser W, Jung E, Erbsloh-Moller B, et al. Validation of the Fibromyalgia Survey Questionnaire within a cross-sectional survey. PLoS One 2012;7(5):e37504.

60. Kim H, Cui J, Frits M, et al. Fibromyalgia and the prediction of two-year changes in functional status in rheumatoid arthritis patients. Arthritis Care Res (Hoboken) 2017;69(12):1871–7.

61. Wolfe F, Walitt B, Rasker JJ, et al. Primary and secondary fibromyalgia are the same: the universality of polysymptomatic distress. J Rheumatol 2019;46(2): 204–12.

62. Wolfe F, Michaud K, Busch RE, et al. Polysymptomatic distress in patients with rheumatoid arthritis: understanding disproportionate response and its spectrum. Arthritis Care Res (Hoboken) 2014;66(10):1465–71.

63. Mayer TG, Neblett R, Cohen H, et al. The development and psychometric validation of the Central Sensitization Inventory. Pain Pract 2012;12(4):276–85.
64. Guler MA, Celik OF, Ayhan FF. The important role of central sensitization in chronic musculoskeletal pain seen in different rheumatic diseases. Clin Rheumatol 2020;39(1):269–74.
65. Freynhagen R, Baron R, Gockel U, et al. painDETECT: a new screening questionnaire to identify neuropathic components in patients with back pain. Curr Med Res Opin 2006;22(10):1911–20.
66. Rifbjerg-Madsen S, Waehrens EE, Danneskiold-Samsoe B, et al. Psychometric properties of the painDETECT questionnaire in rheumatoid arthritis, psoriatic arthritis and spondyloarthritis: Rasch analysis and test-retest reliability. Health Qual Life Outcomes 2017;15(1):110.
67. Rifbjerg-Madsen S, Christensen AW, Boesen M, et al. The course of pain hypersensitivity according to painDETECT in patients with rheumatoid arthritis initiating treatment: results from the prospective FRAME-cohort study. Arthritis Res Ther 2018;20(1):105.
68. Koop SM, ten Klooster PM, Vonkeman HE, et al. Neuropathic-like pain features and cross-sectional associations in rheumatoid arthritis. Arthritis Res Ther 2015; 17:237.
69. Rifbjerg-Madsen S, Christensen AW, Christensen R, et al. Pain and pain mechanisms in patients with inflammatory arthritis: a Danish nationwide cross-sectional DANBIO registry survey. PLoS One 2017;12(7):e0180014.
70. Christensen AW, Rifbjerg-Madsen S, Christensen R, et al. Non-nociceptive pain in rheumatoid arthritis is frequent and affects disease activity estimation: cross-sectional data from the FRAME study. Scand J Rheumatol 2016;45(6):461–9.
71. Salaffi F, Di Carlo M, Carotti M, et al. The effect of neuropathic pain symptoms on remission in patients with early rheumatoid arthritis. Curr Rheumatol Rev 2019; 15(2):154–61.
72. Ten Klooster PM, de Graaf N, Vonkeman HE. Association between pain phenotype and disease activity in rheumatoid arthritis patients: a non-interventional, longitudinal cohort study. Arthritis Res Ther 2019;21(1):257.
73. Neville SJ, Clauw AD, Moser SE, et al. Association between the 2011 fibromyalgia survey criteria and multisite pain sensitivity in knee osteoarthritis. Clin J Pain 2018;34(10):909–17.
74. Hendriks E, Voogt L, Lenoir D, et al. Convergent validity of the Central Sensitization Inventory in chronic whiplash-associated disorders; associations with quantitative sensory testing, pain intensity, fatigue, and psychosocial factors. Pain Med 2020. https://doi.org/10.1093/pm/pnaa276.
75. Cruz-Almeida Y, Fillingim RB. Can quantitative sensory testing move us closer to mechanism-based pain management? Pain Med 2014;15(1):61–72.
76. Pavlakovic G, Petzke F. The role of quantitative sensory testing in the evaluation of musculoskeletal pain conditions. Curr Rheumatol Rep 2010;12(6):455–61.
77. Dhondt W, Willaeys T, Verbruggen LA, et al. Pain threshold in patients with rheumatoid arthritis and effect of manual oscillations. Scand J Rheumatol 1999; 28(2):88–93.
78. Fredriksson L, Alstergren P, Kopp S. Pressure pain thresholds in the craniofacial region of female patients with rheumatoid arthritis. J Orofac Pain 2003;17(4): 326–32.
79. Joharatnam N, McWilliams DF, Wilson D, et al. A cross-sectional study of pain sensitivity, disease-activity assessment, mental health, and fibromyalgia status in rheumatoid arthritis. Arthritis Res Ther 2015;17:11.

80. Lee YC, Bingham CO 3rd, Edwards RR, et al. Association between pain sensitization and disease activity in patients with rheumatoid arthritis: a cross-sectional study. Arthritis Care Res (Hoboken) 2018;70(2):197–204.
81. Lee YC, Chibnik LB, Lu B, et al. The relationship between disease activity, sleep, psychiatric distress and pain sensitivity in rheumatoid arthritis: a cross-sectional study. Arthritis Res Ther 2009;11(5):R160.
82. Gerecz-Simon EM, Tunks ER, Heale JA, et al. Measurement of pain threshold in patients with rheumatoid arthritis, osteoarthritis, ankylosing spondylitis, and healthy controls. Clin Rheumatol 1989;8(4):467–74.
83. Lofgren M, Opava CH, Demmelmaier I, et al. Pain sensitivity at rest and during muscle contraction in persons with rheumatoid arthritis: a substudy within the Physical Activity in Rheumatoid Arthritis 2010 study. Arthritis Res Ther 2018;20(1):48.
84. Heisler AC, Song J, Dunlop DD, et al. Association of pain centralization and patient-reported pain in active rheumatoid arthritis. Arthritis Care Res (Hoboken) 2020;72(8):1122–9.
85. Graven-Nielsen T, Arendt-Nielsen L. Assessment of mechanisms in localized and widespread musculoskeletal pain. Nat Rev Rheumatol 2010;6(10):599–606.
86. Hermans L, Nijs J, Calders P, et al. Influence of morphine and naloxone on pain modulation in rheumatoid arthritis, chronic fatigue syndrome/fibromyalgia, and controls: a double-blind, randomized, placebo-controlled, cross-over study. Pain Pract 2018;18(4):418–30.
87. Vladimirova N, Jespersen A, Bartels EM, et al. Pain sensitisation in women with active rheumatoid arthritis: a comparative cross-sectional study. Arthritis 2015;2015:434109.
88. Heisler AC, Song J, Muhammad LN, et al. Association of dysregulated central pain processing and response to disease-modifying antirheumatic drug therapy in rheumatoid arthritis. Arthritis Rheumatol 2020;72(12):2017–24.
89. Christensen AW, Rifbjerg-Madsen S, Christensen R, et al. Ultrasound Doppler but not temporal summation of pain predicts DAS28 response in rheumatoid arthritis: a prospective cohort study. Rheumatology (Oxford) 2016 Jun;55(6):1091–8. https://doi.org/10.1093/rheumatology/kew034.
90. Damien J, Colloca L, Bellei-Rodriguez CE, et al. Pain modulation: from conditioned pain modulation to placebo and nocebo effects in experimental and clinical pain. Int Rev Neurobiol 2018;139:255–96.
91. Le Bars D. The whole body receptive field of dorsal horn multireceptive neurones. Brain Res Brain Res Rev 2002;40(1–3):29–44.
92. Yarnitsky D, Arendt-Nielsen L, Bouhassira D, et al. Recommendations on terminology and practice of psychophysical DNIC testing. Eur J Pain 2010;14(4):339.
93. Staud R. Abnormal endogenous pain modulation is a shared characteristic of many chronic pain conditions. Expert Rev Neurother 2012;12(5):577–85.
94. Meeus M, Hermans L, Ickmans K, et al. Endogenous pain modulation in response to exercise in patients with rheumatoid arthritis, patients with chronic fatigue syndrome and comorbid fibromyalgia, and healthy controls: a double-blind randomized controlled trial. Pain Pract 2015;15(2):98–106.
95. Meeus M, Ickmans K, Struyf F, et al. Does acetaminophen activate endogenous pain inhibition in chronic fatigue syndrome/fibromyalgia and rheumatoid arthritis? A double-blind randomized controlled cross-over trial. Pain Physician 2013;16(2):E61–70.
96. Jones AK, Huneke NT, Lloyd DM, et al. Role of functional brain imaging in understanding rheumatic pain. Curr Rheumatol Rep 2012;14(6):557–67.

97. Harvey AK, Taylor AM, Wise RG. Imaging pain in arthritis: advances in structural and functional neuroimaging. Curr Pain Headache Rep 2012;16(6):492–501.
98. Wartolowska K, Hough MG, Jenkinson M, et al. Structural changes of the brain in rheumatoid arthritis. Arthritis Rheum 2012;64(2):371–9.
99. Schrepf A, Kaplan CM, Ichesco E, et al. A multi-modal MRI study of the central response to inflammation in rheumatoid arthritis. Nat Commun 2018;9(1):2243.
100. Lee YC, Fine A, Protsenko E, et al. Brain correlates of continuous pain in rheumatoid arthritis as measured by pulsed arterial spin labeling. Arthritis Care Res (Hoboken) 2019;71(2):308–18.
101. Detre JA, Rao H, Wang DJ, et al. Applications of arterial spin labeled MRI in the brain. J Magn Reson Imaging 2012;35(5):1026–37.
102. Sandstrom A, Ellerbrock I, Jensen KB, et al. Altered cerebral pain processing of noxious stimuli from inflamed joints in rheumatoid arthritis: an event-related fMRI study. Brain Behav Immun 2019;81:272–9.
103. Mars RB, Neubert FX, Noonan MP, et al. On the relationship between the "default mode network" and the "social brain". Front Hum Neurosci 2012;6:189.
104. Napadow V, Kim J, Clauw DJ, et al. Decreased intrinsic brain connectivity is associated with reduced clinical pain in fibromyalgia. Arthritis Rheum 2012;64(7):2398–403.
105. Hsiao FJ, Wang SJ, Lin YY, et al. Altered insula-default mode network connectivity in fibromyalgia: a resting-state magnetoencephalographic study. J Headache Pain 2017;18(1):89.
106. Ceko M, Frangos E, Gracely J, et al. Default mode network changes in fibromyalgia patients are largely dependent on current clinical pain. Neuroimage 2020;216:116877.
107. Kaplan CM, Schrepf A, Ichesco E, et al. Association of inflammation with pronociceptive brain connections in rheumatoid arthritis patients with concomitant fibromyalgia. Arthritis Rheumatol 2020;72(1):41–6.
108. Basu N, Kaplan CM, Ichesco E, et al. Neurobiologic features of fibromyalgia are also present among rheumatoid arthritis patients. Arthritis Rheumatol 2018;70(7):1000–7.
109. Rech J, Hess A, Finzel S, et al. Association of brain functional magnetic resonance activity with response to tumor necrosis factor inhibition in rheumatoid arthritis. Arthritis Rheum 2013;65(2):325–33.

Sexual Dimorphism in the Expression of Pain Phenotype in Preclinical Models of Rheumatoid Arthritis

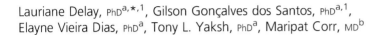

Lauriane Delay, PhD[a],*,[1], Gilson Gonçalves dos Santos, PhD[a],[1],
Elayne Vieira Dias, PhD[a], Tony L. Yaksh, PhD[a], Maripat Corr, MD[b]

KEYWORDS

- Rheumatoid arthritis • Pain • Sexual dimorphism

KEY POINTS

- Rheumatoid arthritis is the most frequent rheumatic disease with a higher prevalence in females than in males.
- Pain is a cardinal symptom of rheumatoid arthritis and strongly impacts patient quality of life.
- Sexual dimorphism in pain processing has been described in the literature since 1988.
- Sexual dimorphism in rheumatoid arthritis has been reported. However, there remains a dearth of studies directly addressing sexual dimorphism in rheumatoid arthritis pain mechanisms.

A BRIEF OVERVIEW OF RHEUMATOID ARTHRITIS

Historically, rheumatoid arthritis (RA) was first described in 1800.[1] It is at present the most frequent chronic inflammatory rheumatic disease.[2] RA prevalence ranges from 0.3% to 1.0% of the population in industrialized countries according to the World Health Organization[3,4] and its incidence increases with the aging of the population.[5,6] This disease is characterized as an autoimmune-mediated inflammatory disease that involves both immunologic activation and inflammatory pathways. Once these pathways are triggered, it results in a self-perpetuating process that leads to joint inflammation, cartilage degradation, bone erosion, and chronic pain.[7] Identification and prognosis of patients with RA have been improved with the recognition of specific anticitrullinated peptide antibodies (ACPA)[8] in addition to rheumatoid factor.[9] Indeed, the detection of anticyclic citrullinated peptides antibodies (anti-CCP) presents with a

[a] Department of Anesthesiology, University of California San Diego, 9500 Gilman Dr., La Jolla, CA 92093, USA; [b] Division of Rheumatology, Allergy and Immunology, University of California San Diego, 9500 Gilman Dr., La Jolla, CA 92093, USA
[1] These authors contributed equally to this work.
* Corresponding author.
E-mail address: ldelay@health.ucsd.edu

Rheum Dis Clin N Am 47 (2021) 245–264
https://doi.org/10.1016/j.rdc.2020.12.006
0889-857X/21/Published by Elsevier Inc.

rheumatic.theclinics.com

98% specificity and are thus considered as useful tools for the diagnosis of rheuma-toid disease.[10] Although the dynamic process of rheumatic disease initiation and pro-gression is not clear, a robust association between genetic,[11–15] epigenetic,[16–21] environmental,[22–29] and immunologic[30–34] components during the development of RA has been demonstrated.

From the genetic perspective, it is well-recognized that RA susceptibility may be strongly linked to family history.[35] The increased prevalence of disease within racial groups has been shown, as in native Americans where prevalence rates of RA of 5% to 7% have been reported.[36] Since the early 1970s, class II human leukocyte an-tigens (HLA) were associated with susceptibility to RA.[37,38] The major HLA susceptible locus associated with RA is *HLA-DRB1*, especially with regard to a specific sequence of amino acids referred to as "the shared epitope" in different *HLA-DRB1* alleles (eg, *01, *04, *10, *14).[39] Specific amino acids at position 11 (eg, Val, Leu, Pro) or 13 (eg, His and Phe) are strongly associated with RA development.[40,41] Other non-HLA genes have been shown to be associated risk factors for developing RA, including *PTPN22, TNF, IL-1B, CRP,* and *CTL4*.[13–15,42] Although these genetic associations with RA sus-ceptibility are robust, there is not a perfect genetic consonance and other factors clearly can contribute to the development of RA. Associated variables that have been strongly implicated in the development of RA include environmental factors, such as cigarette smoking,[22] pollutants (eg, silica),[43] and patient variables (eg, diet),[44] mucosal microbiomes,[28,29,45–47] and sex/gender.[48,49]

Of particular interest in this review is the issue of the sex linkages and the develop-ment and progression of RA. The RA diagnosis in fact presents as a heterogeneous phenotype, the severity and patterns of which are influenced by sex-associated factors. RA is 2 to 5 times more common in women than men, depending on the region in the world.[5,6] In women, RA onset is commonly seen between 30 to 60 years of age, whereas in men, RA often begins later in life.[50] Thus, after the age of 65, the ratio of the incidence in men and women shifts with the predominance occurring in men more than 75 years of age.[49] Although it is not clear which factors drive the sexual dimorphism in patients with RA, comparing clinical data in humans, and preclinical studies in rodents, several hy-potheses have been proposed based on sex hormones[51–53] and immune cells.[54]

PAIN IN RHEUMATOID ARTHRITIS
Model of Phases of Pain in Rheumatoid Arthritis

The mechanisms underlying pain state in the patient with RA represent complex pro-cesses that differ between stages of the disease (**Fig. 1**).[55] The production of autoan-tibodies (eg, rheumatoid factor, ACPA, anti-CarP) starts months to years before the onset of the disease, gradually increasing[56] (dark blue line; see **Fig. 1, ❶**). We now recognize in the early preclinical arthritis phase, patients can suffer from arthralgia (purple line; see **Fig. 1, ❶**) before the development of clinically evident signs, such as palpable synovitis (dotted blue line; see **Fig. 1, ❶**). In the subsequent development of active disease (eg, with clinical signs of joint pathology), patients with RA develop chronic inflammatory joint pain, which display a cyclic waxing and waning (see **Fig. 1, ❷**). These clinical signs may then display some degree of remission after treatment with modern therapies. In remission, pain resolves in some patients (see **Fig. 1, ❸**), but in a significant proportion of patients arthralgia persists[57] (see **Fig. 1, ❹**). More-over, remission is not necessarily associated with declining autoantibody titers and disappearance of autoantibodies remains rare[58] (dotted dark blue line; see **Fig. 1, ❹**). Mechanisms involved in RA pain are also different between stages (for an exten-sive literature on this subject see reviews[55,59–62]).

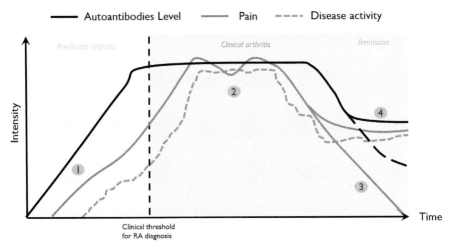

Fig. 1. Pain evolution according to RA disease activity. In RA, pain symptom in patients follows different steps[55]: ❶ in a preclinical stage, patient can develop arthralgia before the onset of the disease potentially associated with an early production of autoantibodies, ❷ after RA diagnostic, in clinical stage, marked by the development of synovitis, pain and disease activity both increase and fluctuate without being entirely correlated each other, ❸ following an effective therapy, pain symptom can decrease in a remission stage, but ❹ in a significant proportion of patients, pain symptoms persist even though the disease activity decreased.

Simplistically, pain processing begins with the activation of nociceptive primary afferents, which innervate the joint.[63] In turn, these nociceptive afferents lead to the activation of second-order neurons in the spinal dorsal horn that project via the ventrolateral long tract to a variety of supraspinal centers in the brain. Some of these projections through the somatosensory thalamus to the somatosensory cortex mediate the so-called sensory discriminative aspect of pain, whereas other projections are through more medial thalamus regions and project to the areas of the limbic forebrain associated with emotion and affect. The consequence is the pain state, which comprises the emotional and affective factors that lead, ultimately, to a protective response.[63,64] Although the acute activation of these circuits normally have a protective role (eg, to evoke for example limb withdrawal), these states, when chronic, become maladaptive. Such chronic pain attributes in RA have a marked prevalence in females.[65–67] However, there is no common pathophysiologic sex-related mechanism shared by all chronic pain conditions; each one can present specific factors that differ between females and males.[68]

Lack of Covariance with Physical Signs and Pain in Rheumatoid Arthritis

An important point to be made in the conceptual summary displayed in **Fig. 1** is that, although joint morphology, pathology, and loss of function primarily underlie the RA diagnosis, pain displays deviations from the expression of the underlying clinically evident pathology for the patient with RA. Of note, this dissociation has particular relevance in that pain is the cardinal symptom of RA that strongly impacts these patients' quality of life.[69] In fact, 75% to 80% of patients with RA in treatment have moderate to severe pain symptoms.[70,71] Only 26% of patients are satisfied with their RA treatment[69] and between 55% and 65% of patients are unsatisfied with their pain management,[70] a priority for patients with RA.[71] It is important to take into account that most of data are obtained from women (75%–90% depending on the study[69,70]). The actual "treat to target" strategy for RA aims to decrease the pathologic changes[72] and thereby to modulate pain. However, joint pain is in fact poorly correlated with the inflammatory state of the patient with RA.[62] Even with optimal regulation of inflammatory cascades, pain has often been shown to be insufficiently controlled.[57] It is well-appreciated that joint pain (arthralgia) often begins before other manifestations of joint inflammation[73,74] and consequently before any diagnosis or the implementation of an RA therapeutic strategy. A further complexity is that, although the RA phenotype involves joint structures (synovia, cartilage, and bones), an autoimmune response outside of the joint is also observed and is usually associated with other pathologies, such as rheumatoid nodules, lymphatic vessel tumefaction, pleuritis, and cardiovascular or ocular manifestations.[75] These observations have led to an appreciation that pain arising in association with RA may reflect parallel processes that may be influenced by the variables that are associated with the physical manifestation of RA and particularly given the role played by sex.

Covariance of Antibodies with Pain and Dissociation from Joint Manifestations

As presented in conceptual summary in **Fig. 1**, arthralgia can in fact be reported months to years before the actual onset of clinically identified disease. It is now appreciated that this onset of arthralgia may occur concurrently with the expression of autoantibodies (ie, rheumatoid factor,[76] ACPA,[77–79] anti-CarP,[80–82] and anti-MAA[83,84]). These autoantibodies can be detectable in patients reporting predisease arthralgias and may be associated with persistent arthralgia during remission. Recently, a direct link between ACPA isolated from patients with RA and pain development in mice has been described[85] and was felt to mechanistically involve chemokine production by osteoclasts.[86] Phenotypic changes of in the Fc portion of antibodies, such as galactosylation, fucosylation, or sialylation, could be involved in the proinflammatory profile acquisition and certainly pronociceptive.[87–90] In addition to autoantibodies, RA is marked by an early alteration of cytokines and chemokines levels, such as IL-5 or IL-17A,[90–93] which are directly able to sensitize the nociceptor.[63]

As indicated in **Fig. 1**, during the clinical stage, synovitis development induces a chronic joint pain marked by peripheral and central sensitization initially induced by immune cells in RA.[55] It is interesting to note that a comorbid condition, fibromyalgia, reflects a chronic widespread pain associated with tenderness, sleep disturbance, and psychiatric distress in the absence of clinical signs of inflammation. This condition affects around 14% to 20% of patients with RA, with a higher prevalence in women.[94,95]

PRECLINICAL MODELS AND SEXUAL DIMORPHISM IN THE PAIN PHENOTYPE OF RHEUMATOID ARTHRITIS

Given the complexities of pain in different stages of arthritis, research efforts have focused on drawing parallels between sex differences observed in RA pathophysiology and sex differences underlying the pain phenotype observed clinically and in preclinical models of RA.

Use of Rodent Models in Arthritis Studies to Study the Role of Sex

Pioneering studies on the sexual dimorphism of pain expression began to emerge around 1988, when Bodnar and associates[96,97] demonstrated sex differences in basal nociceptive thresholds in rodents that seemed to be modulated by sex hormones. In particular, a large number of publications came in the mid-1990s and drew considerable attention to the topic.[66,68,98] Previously, most preclinical studies traditionally used males as subjects and the sex-related differences in pain and their mechanisms were not explored widely. In 2016, the National Institutes of Health initiated a policy requiring preclinical research to use males and females in supported research. Currently, it is clear that males and females do not manifest the same pain experience, showing different physiologic and behaviorally defined pain responses.[67–74] As reviewed elsewhere in this article, overall, females, in preclinical models, often present a lower threshold and or a heightened pain response than that observed in males.[99–101]

Preclinical animal models of RA have been used to understand the pain phenotype and response to analgesic drugs during development and maintenance of RA and can be used to concurrently examine male and female rodents. Here we introduce animal models of RA that have been used to understand sexual dimorphism in the RA pain phenotype and studies directly addressing different hypotheses in relation to pain mechanisms at the levels of primary afferent neurons, dorsal root ganglia (DRG) and trigeminal ganglia, the dorsal horn of the spinal cord, and supraspinal structures.

Several preclinical models have been widely used to understand pain processing and sexual dimorphism in RA (for review see[61,102,103]). Broadly speaking, these models represent the induction of monoarthritis or polyarthritis with time-dependent changes in the joint morphology (eg, synovial lesions, bone resorption, and cartilage destruction), in the inflammatory phenotype (eg, synovial inflammation, infiltration of immune cells), and in the development of pronounced and ongoing pain and changes in behavior, including pain evoked behaviors (eg, mechanical and thermal thresholds), pain-suppressed behaviors (eg, feeding, mating, and locomotor activity), and operant conditioning (eg, conditioned place preference).[102] As will be noted, in comparison with the immunization model, collagen-induced arthritis, the collagen-antibody–induced arthritis (CAIA), and K/BxN models present over time evidence of evolving pain phenotypes.[104] A brief description of these models is presented.

i. The complete Freud's adjuvant (CFA) generated by an intradermal injection[105] (polyarthritis) or an intra-articular injection of CFA (monoarthritis).[106,107] This model is mediated by the innate immune system and leads to the infiltration of inflammatory cells, synovial hypertrophy, and joint alterations, as well as inflammatory response in the viscera, skin, and muscle. These rodents develop hypersensitivity to innocuous stimuli with an immediate onset (<24 hours) and persisting for weeks.

ii. The collagen-induced arthritis model, which is induced by intradermal injection(s) of type II collagen that activate the adaptive immune system and the production of anticollagen II antibodies. This model of polyarthritis leads to a breach of self-tolerance, T- and B-cell activity and activation of anticartilage immunity.[108] In this model, animals develop hypersensitivity at the onset of the disease (within the second week) that persists for at least 28 days.

iii. The CAIA model is induced by an intraperitoneal or intravenous injection of a cocktail of anticollagen II antibodies followed by an intraperitoneal injection of lipopolysaccharide to synchronize the onset of inflammation. The CAIA model of polyarthritis does not involve T and B cells, but directly uses antibodies against joint-specific epitopes, leading to synovial inflammation, the infiltration of immune cells, and the destruction of bone and cartilage. In this model, mechanical hypersensitivity precedes the inflammatory phase and persists for 3 to 4 months, even after the resolution of inflammation.[61]

iv. The K/BxN passive serum transfer model of polyarthritis is induced by the intraperitoneal injection(s) of sera from KRN-NOD (K/BxN) transgenic mice that demonstrate an inflammatory arthritis phenotype that begins shortly after weaning and continues unabated into adulthood.[109] The serum from the transgenic K/BxN mice contains antibodies directed against glucose-6-phosphate isomerase and associated immune complexes, leading to synovial inflammation, the infiltration of immune cells, and the destruction of bone and cartilage. This model is characterized by a biphasic period where tactile and cold allodynia are observed very early after the delivery of the K/BxN serum.[110] The clinical signs (eg, joint swelling, erythema) resolve and, of note, the allodynia persists unabated. As noted in **Table 1**, the early phase displays an inflammatory analgesic pharmacology, whereas the late phase seems to represent an analgesic pharmacology of a neuropathic state.

As shown in **Table 1**, in the models as described elsewhere in this article, a sexual dimorphism for arthritis score, pain phenotype, neuraxial changes, and response to treatment has been a focus of limited research to date with direct comparisons. Regarding inflammation, females exhibited a higher arthritis score in CFA rats and female rats with collagen-induced arthritis had a greater susceptibility than males, whereas in the CAIA and K/BxN passive transfer models, no difference was observed in arthritis development between sexes (in mice). For the pain phenotype, a sexual dimorphism was observed in female CFA rats that presented a lower evoked paw pressure threshold, whereas there were no differences in the collagen-induced arthritis male and female rats. In contrast, female K/BxN passive serum transfer mice showed a resolution in both paw inflammation and evoked mechanical allodynia pain phenotype in the late phase, whereas males presented a postinflammatory and long-lasting allodynia.

Major sexual dimorphism was observed in the molecular mechanism of pain processing; indeed, in the CAIA and K/BxN models. Female mice showed a spinal microglia (ie, the ionized calcium binding adaptor molecule 1 marker) activation in early and late phases and astrocyte activation (ie, the glial fibrillary acidic protein marker) only in the late phase. Interestingly, K/BxN male mice presented only microglial activation in the late phase and no significant astrocyte activation. In the CAIA model, both males and females showed an increase of spinal calcitonin gene-related peptide and substance P, key neuropeptides involved in central sensitization playing a role in the development and maintenance of hyperalgesia,[114] but spinal galanin, a neuropeptide known to be involved in neuropathic pain, was only increased in males in the late phase of CAIA. In the K/BxN model, both males and females show an enhanced expression of tumor necrosis factor in the spinal cord at the peak of paw inflammation. However, also in the spinal cord females showed enhanced IL-10 messenger RNA (mRNA) and in the late phase increased type I interferon-beta mRNA expression compared with male mice. These protein and mRNA markers are leading to our cellular and molecular understanding of the sex differences seen in the pain phenotypes in arthritis.

In addition to the differences in the biomarkers of pain, there were sex differences in the responses to pharmacologic treatments. In the CFA model, opioid agonists (eg, morphine, butorphanol, oxycodone, and loperamide) were more potent in males than in females. Intrathecal administration of glial inhibitors using minocycline or pentoxifylline were only effective in male CIAI mice, highlighting a prominent role for microglia in male pain processing. Intrathecal injections also demonstrated that pain modulation was largely at the spinal cord/DRG level in the K/BxN model. In the K/BxN mice, intrathecal injection of anti-tumor necrosis factor antibodies transiently reduced pain as did the injections of interferon-ß. Neither single agent was effective

Table 1
Sexual differences in preclinical models of inflammatory arthritis

Model	Species	Arthritis Score	Pain Phenotype	Neuraxial Changes	Response to Treatment	References
CFA	Lewis rats	♀>♂	♀>♂	Not investigated	Morphine 5 times more potent in ♂-treated CFA vs ♀ Butorphanol 62 times more potent in ♂-treated CFA vs ♀ Oxycodone greater % of antihyperalgesia in ♂-treated CFA vs ♀ Loperamide 4 times more potent in ♂-treated CFA vs ♀Naloxone ♀ = ♂	Cook & Nickerson,[105] 2005
CIA	Lewis rats Dark agouti rats Spragues Dawley rats	♀>♂	♀ = ♂	Not investigated	Tropomyosin receptor kinase A inhibitor AR786 reduced pain behavior - data for ♀ and ♂ were not separated	Ashraf et al,[111] 2016; Dimitrijević et al,[54] 2020
CAIA	Balb/c mice CBA mice C57BL/6 mice	♀ = ♂	♀ = ♂	In the spinal dorsal horn: ↗Ibal immunoreactivity early and late phase ♀ = ♂ ↗GFAP late phase ♀ = ♂ ↗Galanin late phase only in ♂	Minocycline and pentoxifylline reversed mechanical hypersensitivity in the late phase only in ♂	Fernandez-Zafra et al,[112] 2019
K/BxN	C57BL/6 mice	♀ = ♂	Early phase ♀ = ♂ Late phase ♀<♂	In the spinal cord: mRNA TNF ♀~♂ mRNA IL-10 ♀>♂ mRNA interferon-β ♀>♂ In the spinal dorsal horn: ↗Ibal early and late phase in ♀ but only late phase for ♂ ↗GFAP late phase only in ♀	♂anti-TNF + interferon-β in the early phase reduced allodynia for at least 7 d	Woller et al,[113] 2019

Abbreviations: ♀, female; ♂, male; CFA, complete Freud adjuvant; CIA, collagen-induced arthritis; CAIA, collagen antibody-induced arthritis; K/BxN, K/BxN serum transfer; GFP, glial fibrillary acidic protein; TNF, tumor necrosis factor.

in the long term; however, 2 injections with both agents permanently reversed the pain phenotype in male mice. This result suggested that the spontaneous biologic advantage of self-remitting pain in female mice could be phenocopied with therapeutic injections of biologic agents at the anatomic level of the difference between male and female pain mechanisms (in this case the intrathecal space).

The Role of Sex Hormones

Sexual dimorphism in the pain experience is probably mostly defined by sex hormones. Although the effect of these hormones on pain is complex and not yet completely understood, it is well-known that sex hormones influence both peripheral and central nervous system pathways by modulating neuronal activity.[115] Considering sex hormones in patients with RA, it is well-known that, during pregnancy, circulating steroid hormones (ie, estrogen, progesterone, and cortisol) seem to directly or indirectly suppress synovial inflammation inhibiting the maternal immune system and inducing an immune tolerance.[51] Moreover, postpartum, breastfeeding is associated with a lower risk of RA[52] and the production of prolactin that has immunomodulatory properties.[116] Furthermore, RA is more frequently observed after menopause and menopause at a young age ($\leq$45 years old) is a risk factor for RA.[53] Some studies also demonstrated a protective effect of progesterone receptor signaling in mice[117] and androgen may also protect against RA development in humans.[118] Conversely, androgen deprivation therapy[119] or hypogonadism[120] increases the risk of RA in men. Therefore, a sexual dimorphism in the expression of pain phenotype in RA is undoubtedly associated, in part, by sex hormones.

Hormonal Receptors on Neurons

Androgen receptors (AR) are expressed in DRG sensory neurons and one-half of AR-positive neurons were nociceptive afferents[121]; some studies have demonstrated the involvement of testosterone in pain modulation.[122–125] It has been shown that primary afferents also express estrogen receptors (ERα and ERβ).[126,127] Preclinical models have shown that ERα expression seems to be restricted to nociceptive afferents whereas ERβ is more widely distributed.[128] It has been demonstrated that ERs can play a role in the control of peripheral nociceptive signaling by interacting with purinergic, P2X3, and transient receptor potential vanilloide 1 receptors in nociceptive afferent neurons.[127,129–133] The expression of both P2X3 and transient receptor potential vanilloide 1 receptors was significantly reduced in female ERs (ERα and ERβ) knockout mice compared with the expression in female wild type mice. Ma and colleagues[130] demonstrated that ovariectomized female rats had an increase of P2X3 expression in DRG neurons followed by a higher mechanical sensitivity, which were reversed by estrogen replacement. In contrast, mechanical sensitivity and P2X3 expression did not change in the DRG of orchiectomized male rats, evidencing the relation between estrogen and P2X3 expression in nociceptive afferents. Because P2X3 receptors are expressed in the fibers innervating joints, this relation between estrogen and P2X3 receptors might explain, at least in part, the sex differences in pain observed in RA.

In addition, estrogen can also mediate the sex-related differences in substance P release[134] and in the expression of both nerve growth factor and its high-affinity receptor tropomyosin receptor kinase A in DRG neurons.[135–137] Substance P expression is altered in the joint and dorsal horn of animals with arthritis.[138,139] Nerve growth factor and its receptor are involved in pain[140] and rheumatic diseases.[141] Calcitonin gene-related peptide expression in DRG neurons also undergoes an estrogen influence.[142] Therefore, the effects of estrogen on nociceptive neurons may also be contributing to the sexual dimorphism in the pain phenotype of RA. However, studies are needed comparing the female and male pain phenotypes and their nociceptive afferent proteomic profiles. This need is more pronounced when a specific condition is considered. Sensory afferent neurons also express prolactin receptors, which modulate neuronal activity majorly in females.[143] Patil and colleagues[143] have shown that prolactin receptor mRNA was expressed equally in female and male peptidergic nociceptors and central terminals; however, prolactin protein was found only in females, and, in turn, prolactin-induced excitability was detected only in female DRG neurons. Strikingly, in patients with RA, both males and females, increased serum levels of prolactin cooperates with other proinflammatory stimuli to activate macrophages,[144] but the clinical significance of prolactin to RA pathogenesis remains unclear. Taking into account these recent data in the literature, it is plausible that, during RA development, primary afferent neurons could play a role in sexual dimorphism of the RA pain phenotype.

Sex Differences in Transcription at the Dorsal Root Ganglion

The sexual dimorphism in response to a noxious stimulus can involve differences at the level of primary afferent neurons, dorsal root and trigeminal ganglia, dorsal horn of the spinal cord and supraspinal structures. DRG and trigeminal ganglia primary afferent neurons have been found as possible source of mechanistic diversity that causes sex differences in pain.[143,145] In fact, studies suggested sex-related differences in the sensory neuron transcriptome. A transcriptomic analysis of DRG shows that prostaglandin D synthase, an enzyme involved in prostaglandins E2 production is upregulated in female neurons.[143,145] Prostaglandins E2 is well-known to be involved in pain processing by inducing neuronal sensitization. Indeed, cyclo-oxygenase inhibitors have been widely used in pain management. Importantly, studies in rodent arthritis models have described decreased inflammation in cyclo-oxygenase–deficient mice in females, but not in males.[146] However, in the same study, pain and sexual dimorphism were not analyzed.

Sex Differences in Microglia and Macrophages

The sensory afferent neuron forms an excitatory synapse with second-order neurons in the dorsal horn of the dorsal spinal cord to initiate transmission in the central nervous system. A sexual dimorphism in pain processing in the spinal cord has been described in the literature,[67,147] including in animal models of RA (see **Table 1**). Mogil and colleagues have shown that hypersensitivity in inflammatory and neuropathic pain conditions in mice, can be attributed to distinct immune cell types: microglia in males and T cells in females.[148,149] Corroborating this finding, the response to intrathecal administration of glial inhibitors are only effective in males and not in females in CAIA mice[112] (see **Table 1**) and reinforced a sex difference in pain neuraxial mechanisms. The purinergic receptor P2X4 is known to play key roles in inflammatory response[150] and is involved in a sex-dependent manner in various pain conditions.[151] In neuropathic pain, a male-specific upregulation of P2X4R has been shown[148] and an inhibition of spinal P2X4R attenuates pain hypersensitivity in males but not females mice,[152] which raises the questions of whether microglial purinergic receptors could be involved in pain and sexual dimorphism in RA.

Sex Differences in Pain Processing by the Brain

Other than DRGs or spinal cord changes, supraspinal structures involved with high-order functions, such as anxiety, depression, and cognition, are critical component for pain processing.[63] There is a sex-related difference in brain structures involved in pain perception and modulation that can be explained, at least in part, by sex-hormones. Periaqueductal gray neurons, which project to the rostral ventral medulla and constituting the primary descending pathway of pain inhibition, express sex hormone receptors. AR and ERα immunoreactive neurons were widely distributed in the caudal periaqueductal gray neurons of male rats. Females had significantly fewer AR-positive neurons, although the quantity of ERα was comparable between the sexes.[153] A preclinical study showed that rostral anterior cingulate cortex, an important brain structure involved in pain affect, is also modulated by estrogen via ER.[154] Considering deep tissue pain in humans, brain imaging studies showed complex brain networks involved in sensory and affective aspects of pain. Under many chronic pain conditions, it was observed greater anterior cingulate cortex activation in females and insular cortex activation in males.[155] This sexual dimorphism of brain areas activation might contribute to different pain-related responses, which could require different treatment based on sex/gender differences. Although sex hormones have been suggested as key drivers of the sexual dimorphism observed in the expression of pain, an important sociocultural component must be also taking into account to explain the difference of pain experience in humans.

SUMMARY AND FUTURE DIRECTIONS

Epidemiologic and clinical findings demonstrate sex differences in several pain conditions, with women at higher risk of developing chronic pain. The central processing of pain information involving higher order neural functions can explain, at least in part, the sex-related differences in pain experienced by patients with RA. However, there is a dearth in the literature of studies directly addressing sex-associated differences and behavior in rodent models of inflammatory pain. As highlighted by Krock and colleagues,[104] nearly 50% of studies focused on pain-like behavior in arthritis were conducted only in male rodents. This observation reinforced that female and especially female/male comparisons in arthritis pain research are still needed. Although RA is an area of intense study, a single rodent model does not fully recapitulate disease. However, current models have been a useful tool to understand the pathophysiology and new targets to treat RA. Therefore, investigations with males and females are needed to advance our understanding of which components of the inflammatory processes that generate pain are subject to sex dimorphisms.

Therapies like nonsteroidal anti-inflammatory drugs have been used to treat pain in RA and in preclinical models of RA.[110,156] However, is important to note that studies suggest a neuropathic phenotype in RA-associated pain,[110,157] which would not be adequately treated by NSAIDs. Therefore, examining available treatments used to treat neuropathic pain might be valuable in addressing RA-associated pain. Strikingly, a sexual dimorphism has been seen when it comes to pain management in some animal models.[158] This finding highlights the necessity for understanding the phenotype of arthritis in both males and females to direct an effective treatment. It is noteworthy that, in parallel to biological factors, psychosocial and cultural factors contribute strongly to sexual dimorphism of pain perception in patients,[159–164] and consequently their response to therapy.

In conclusion, several animal models of RA have contributed our understanding of the pathogenesis of RA and therapeutic management. However, we still need to navigate through RA under a pain perspective, correlating key factors of RA that have not been tested in the pain context and considering both sexes.

CLINICS CARE POINTS

- Inflammatory joint pain exemplified in rheumatoid arthritis is regulated by different processes in males and females.

- Some, but not all, of the sex differences in pain processing are associated with sex hormones and their receptors.

- Sexual dimorphism in pain processing may also lead to sex differences in response to treatment and therapies should be evaluated for differences in efficacy in males and females.

DISCLOSURE

The authors receive grant support from United States, NIH/NINDS 1 R01 NS099338 and 1 R01 NS102432-01.

REFERENCES

1. Tsoucalas G, Sgantzos M. Primary Asthenic gout by Augustin-Jacob Landre-Beauvais in 1800: is this the first description of rheumatoid arthritis? Mediterr J Rheumatol 2017;28(4):223–6.

2. Jokar M, Jokar M. Prevalence of inflammatory rheumatic diseases in a rheumatologic outpatient clinic: analysis of 12626 cases. Rheumatol Res 2018;3(1): 21–7 https://doi.org/10.22631/rr.2017.69997.1037.

3. WHO scientific group on the burden of musculoskeletal conditions at the start of the new millennium. The burden of musculoskeletal conditions at the start of the new millennium. World Health Organ Tech Rep Ser. 2003;919:i-x, 1-218, back cover. Available at: http://www.ncbi.nlm.nih.gov/pubmed/14679827. Accessed January 15, 2018.

4. Minichiello E, Semerano L, Boissier MC. Incidence, prévalence et sévérité de la polyarthrite rhumatoïde au XXIe siècle. Rev du Rhum Monogr 2017;84(4): 303–10. https://doi.org/10.1016/j.monrhu.2017.07.002.

5. Cross M, Smith E, Hoy D, et al. The global burden of rheumatoid arthritis: estimates from the global burden of disease 2010 study. Ann Rheum Dis 2014; 73(7):1316–22.

6. Rudan I, Sidhu S, Papana A, et al. Prevalence of rheumatoid arthritis in low- and middle-income countries: a systematic review and analysis. J Glob Health 2015; 5(1):010409.

7. Smolen JS, Aletaha D, Barton A, et al. Rheumatoid arthritis. Nat Rev Dis Primers 2018;4:18001.

8. Aletaha D, Neogi T, Silman AJ, et al. 2010 Rheumatoid arthritis classification criteria: an American college of rheumatology/European league against rheumatism collaborative initiative. Arthritis Rheum 2010;62(9):2569–81.

9. van Zanten A, Arends S, Roozendaal C, et al. Presence of anticitrullinated protein antibodies in a large population-based cohort from the Netherlands. Ann Rheum Dis 2017;76(7):1184–90.

10. Musset L, Ghillani-Dalbin P. La polyarthrite rhumatoïde: Apport de la biologie au diagnostic et au suivi thérapeutique. Immuno-Analyse Biol Spec 2013;28(5–6): 281–6. https://doi.org/10.1016/j.immbio.2013.05.001.

11. Frisell T, Holmqvist M, Källberg H, et al. Familial risks and heritability of rheumatoid arthritis: role of rheumatoid factor/anti-citrullinated protein antibody status, number and type of affected relatives, sex, and age. Arthritis Rheum 2013; 65(11):2773–82.

12. Frisell T, Saevarsdottir S, Askling J. Family history of rheumatoid arthritis: an old concept with new developments. Nat Rev Rheumatol 2016;12(6):335–43.
13. Viatte S, Barton A. Genetics of rheumatoid arthritis susceptibility, severity, and treatment response. Semin Immunopathol 2017;39(4):395–408.
14. Okada Y, Wu D, Trynka G, et al. Genetics of rheumatoid arthritis contributes to biology and drug discovery. Nature 2014;506(7488):376–81.
15. Angelotti F, Parma A, Cafaro G, et al. One year in review 2017: pathogenesis of rheumatoid arthritis. Clin Exp Rheumatol 2017;35(3):0368–78. Available at: http://www.ncbi.nlm.nih.gov/pubmed/28631608. Accessed August 1, 2017.
16. Richez C, Barnetche T, Schaeverbeke T, Truchetet ME. La polyarthrite rhumatoïde: une physiopathologie mieux connue? Rev du Rhum Monogr 2017; 84(4):311–7. https://doi.org/10.1016/j.monrhu.2017.07.006.
17. Ai R, Hammaker D, Boyle DL, et al. Joint-specific DNA methylation and transcriptome signatures in rheumatoid arthritis identify distinct pathogenic processes. Nat Commun 2016;7:11849.
18. Hammaker D, Firestein GS. Epigenetics of inflammatory arthritis. Curr Opin Rheumatol 2018;30(2):188–96.
19. Doody KM, Bottini N, Firestein GS. Epigenetic alterations in rheumatoid arthritis fibroblast-like synoviocytes. Epigenomics 2017;9(4):479–92.
20. Grabiec AM, Korchynskyi O, Tak PP, et al. Histone deacetylase inhibitors suppress rheumatoid arthritis fibroblast-like synoviocytc and macrophage IL-6 production by accelerating mRNA decay. Ann Rheum Dis 2012;71(3):424–31.
21. Mu N, Gu J, Huang T, et al. A novel NF-κB/YY1/microRNA-10a regulatory circuit in fibroblast-like synoviocytes regulates inflammation in rheumatoid arthritis. Sci Rep 2016;6(1):20059.
22. Chang K, Yang SM, Kim SH, et al. Smoking and rheumatoid arthritis. Int J Mol Sci 2014;15(12):22279–95.
23. Costenbader KH, Feskanich D, Mandl LA, et al. Smoking intensity, duration, and cessation, and the risk of rheumatoid arthritis in women. Am J Med 2006;119(6): 503.e1–9.
24. Di Giuseppe D, Orsini N, Alfredsson L, et al. Cigarette smoking and smoking cessation in relation to risk of rheumatoid arthritis in women. Arthritis Res Ther 2013;15(2):R56.
25. Hedström AK, Stawiarz L, Klareskog L, et al. Smoking and susceptibility to rheumatoid arthritis in a Swedish population-based case–control study. Eur J Epidemiol 2018. https://doi.org/10.1007/s10654-018-0360-5.
26. Källberg H, Ding B, Padyukov L, et al. Smoking is a major preventable risk factor for rheumatoid arthritis: estimations of risks after various exposures to cigarette smoke. Ann Rheum Dis 2011;70(3):508–11.
27. Lee S-Y, Lee SH, Jhun J, et al. A combination with probiotic complex, zinc, and coenzyme Q10 attenuates autoimmune arthritis by regulation of Th17/Treg balance. J Med Food 2018;21(1):39–46.
28. Zhang X, Zhang D, Jia H, et al. The oral and gut microbiomes are perturbed in rheumatoid arthritis and partly normalized after treatment. Nat Med 2015;21(8): 895–905.
29. Scher JU, Sczesnak A, Longman RS, et al. Expansion of intestinal Prevotella copri correlates with enhanced susceptibility to arthritis. Elife 2013;2:e01202.
30. Khandpur R, Carmona-Rivera C, Vivekanandan-Giri A, et al. NETs are a source of citrullinated autoantigens and stimulate inflammatory responses in rheumatoid arthritis. Sci Transl Med 2013;5(178):178ra40.

31. Sur Chowdhury C, Giaglis S, Walker UA, et al. Enhanced neutrophil extracellular trap generation in rheumatoid arthritis: analysis of underlying signal transduction pathways and potential diagnostic utility. Arthritis Res Ther 2014;16(3): R122.
32. Berthelot J-M, Le Goff B, Neel A, et al. NETose: au carrefour des polyarthrites rhumatoïdes, lupus et vascularites. Rev Rhum 2017;84(4):274–81.
33. Demoruelle MK, Harrall KK, Ho L, et al. Anti-citrullinated protein antibodies are associated with neutrophil extracellular traps in the sputum in relatives of rheumatoid arthritis patients. Arthritis Rheumatol 2017;69(6):1165–75.
34. van Loosdregt J, Rossetti M, Spreafico R, et al. Increased autophagy in CD4 + T cells of rheumatoid arthritis patients results in T-cell hyperactivation and apoptosis resistance. Eur J Immunol 2016;46(12):2862–70.
35. Sparks JA, Iversen MD, Miller Kroouze R, et al. Personalized risk estimator for rheumatoid arthritis (PRE-RA) family study: rationale and design for a randomized controlled trial evaluating rheumatoid arthritis risk education to first-degree relatives. Contemp Clin Trials 2014;39(1):145–57.
36. Ferucci ED, Templin DW, Lanier AP. Rheumatoid arthritis in American Indians and Alaska natives: a review of the literature. Semin Arthritis Rheum 2005; 34(4):662–7.
37. McMichael AJ, Sasazuki T, McDevitt HO, et al. Increased frequency of HLA-Cw3 and HLA-Dw4 in rheumatoid arthritis. Arthritis Rheum 1977;20(5):1037–42.
38. Stastny P. Association of the B-Cell Alloantigen DRw4 with rheumatoid arthritis. N Engl J Med 1970;298(10).869–71.
39. Gregersen PK, Silver J, Winchester RJ. The shared epitope hypothesis. An approach to understanding the molecular genetics of susceptibility to rheumatoid arthritis. Arthritis Rheum 1987;30(11):1205–13. Available at: http://www.ncbi.nlm.nih.gov/pubmed/2446635. Accessed March 5, 2018.
40. Raychaudhuri S, Sandor C, Stahl EA, et al. Five amino acids in three HLA proteins explain most of the association between MHC and seropositive rheumatoid arthritis. Nat Genet 2012;44(3):291–6.
41. Ling SF, Viatte S, Lunt M, et al. HLA-DRB1 amino acid positions 11/13, 71, and 74 are associated with inflammation level, disease activity, and the health assessment questionnaire score in patients with inflammatory polyarthritis. Arthritis Rheumatol 2016;68(11):2618–28.
42. Piñero J, Queralt-Rosinach N, Bravo À, et al. DisGeNET: a discovery platform for the dynamical exploration of human diseases and their genes. Database (Oxford) 2015;2015:bav028.
43. Stolt P, Källberg H, Lundberg I, et al. Silica exposure is associated with increased risk of developing rheumatoid arthritis: results from the Swedish EIRA study. Ann Rheum Dis 2005;64(4):582–6.
44. Deane KD, Demoruelle MK, Kelmenson LB, et al. Genetic and environmental risk factors for rheumatoid arthritis. Best Pract Res Clin Rheumatol 2017; 31(1):3–18.
45. Vaahtovuo J, MUNUKKA E, KORKEAMÄKI M, et al. Fecal Microbiota in Early Rheumatoid Arthritis. J Rheumatol 2008;35(8). Available at: http://www.jrheum.org/content/35/8/1500.long. Accessed January 19, 2018.
46. Gul'neva MI, Noskov SM. Colonic microbial biocenosis in rheumatoid arthritis. Klin Med (Mosk) 2011;89(4):45–8. Available at: http://www.ncbi.nlm.nih.gov/pubmed/21932563. Accessed January 19, 2018.
47. Liu X, Zou Q, Zeng B, et al. Analysis of fecal lactobacillus community structure in patients with early rheumatoid arthritis. Curr Microbiol 2013;67(2):170–6.

48. Khalifa O, Pers YM, Ferreira R, et al. X-linked miRNAs associated with gender differences in rheumatoid arthritis. Int J Mol Sci 2016;17(11). https://doi.org/10.3390/ijms17111852.

49. Ortona E, Pierdominici M, Maseli A, et al. Sex-based differences in autoimmune diseases. Ann Ist Super Sanita 2016;52(2):205–12.

50. Jawaheer D, Lum RF, Gregersen PK, et al. Influence of male sex on disease phenotype in familial rheumatoid arthritis. Arthritis Rheum 2006;54(10):3087–94.

51. Hughes GC, Choubey D. Modulation of autoimmune rheumatic diseases by oestrogen and progesterone. Nat Rev Rheumatol 2014;10(12):740–51.

52. Chen H, Wang J, Zhou W, et al. Breastfeeding and risk of rheumatoid arthritis: a systematic review and metaanalysis. J Rheumatol 2015;42(9):1563–9.

53. Alpízar-Rodríguez D, Pluchino N, Canny G, Gabay C, Finckh A. The role of female hormonal factors in the development of rheumatoid arthritis. Rheumatol (United Kingdom) 2017;56(8):1254–63. https://doi.org/10.1093/rheumatology/kew318.

54. Dimitrijević M, Arsenović-Ranin N, Kosec D, et al. Sex differences in Tfh cell help to B cells contribute to sexual dimorphism in severity of rat collagen-induced arthritis. Sci Rep 2020;10(1). https://doi.org/10.1038/s41598-020-58127-y.

55. McWilliams DF, Walsh DA. Pain mechanisms in rheumatoid arthritis. Suppl 1(5). Clin Exp Rheumatol 2017;35:94–101. Available at: http://www.ncbi.nlm.nih.gov/pubmed/28967354. Accessed July 3, 2018.

56. van Delft MAM, Huizinga TWJ. An overview of autoantibodies in rheumatoid arthritis. J Autoimmun 2020;110:102392.

57. Lee YC, Cui J, Lu B, et al. Pain persists in DAS28 rheumatoid arthritis remission but not in ACR/EULAR remission: a longitudinal observational study. Arthritis Res Ther 2011;13(3):R83.

58. Boeters DM, Burgers LE, Toes REM, et al. Does immunological remission, defined as disappearance of autoantibodies, occur with current treatment strategies? A long-term follow-up study in rheumatoid arthritis patients who achieved sustained DMARD-free status. Ann Rheum Dis 2019;78(11):1497–504.

59. Walsh DA, McWilliams DF. Mechanisms, impact and management of pain in rheumatoid arthritis. Nat Rev Rheumatol 2014;10(10):581–92.

60. Catrina AI, Svensson CI, Malmström V, et al. Mechanisms leading from systemic autoimmunity to joint-specific disease in rheumatoid arthritis. Nat Rev Rheumatol 2017;13(2):79–86.

61. Bas DB, Su J, Wigerblad G, et al. Pain in rheumatoid arthritis: models and mechanisms. Pain Manag 2016;6(3):265–84.

62. Sarzi-Puttini P, Salaffi F, Di Franco M, et al. Pain in rheumatoid arthritis: a critical review. Reumatismo 2014;66(1):18–27. Available at: http://www.ncbi.nlm.nih.gov/pubmed/24938192. Accessed April 27, 2018.

63. Gonçalves dos Santos G, Delay L, Yaksh TL, et al. Neuraxial cytokines in pain states. Front Immunol 2020;10:3061.

64. Yaksh TL, Hunt MA, dos Santos GG. Development of new analgesics: an answer to opioid epidemic. Trends Pharmacol Sci 2018;39(12):1000–2.

65. Torrance N, Smith BH, Bennett MI, et al. The epidemiology of chronic pain of predominantly neuropathic origin. results from a general population survey. J Pain 2006;7(4):281–9.

66. Fillingim RB, King CD, Ribeiro-Dasilva MC, et al. Sex, gender, and pain: a review of recent clinical and experimental findings. J Pain 2009;10(5):447–85.

67. Mapplebeck JCS, Beggs S, Salter MW. Sex differences in pain: a tale of two immune cells. Pain 2016;157:S2–6.

68. Aloisi AM. Why we still need to speak about sex differences and sex hormones in pain. Pain Ther 2017;6(2):111–4.
69. Radawski C, Genovese MC, Hauber B, et al. Patient perceptions of unmet medical need in rheumatoid arthritis: a cross-sectional survey in the USA. Rheumatol Ther 2019;6(3):461–71.
70. Taylor P, Manger B, Alvaro-Gracia J, et al. Patient perceptions concerning pain management in the treatment of rheumatoid arthritis. J Int Med Res 2010;38(4):1213–24.
71. Heiberg T, Kvien TK. Preferences for improved health examined in 1,024 patients with rheumatoid arthritis: pain has highest priority. Arthritis Rheum 2002;47(4):391–7.
72. Bergstra SA, Allaart CF. What is the optimal target for treat-to-target strategies in rheumatoid arthritis? Curr Opin Rheumatol 2018;1. https://doi.org/10.1097/BOR.0000000000000484.
73. van Baarsen LGM, de Hair MJH, Ramwadhdoebe TH, et al. The cellular composition of lymph nodes in the earliest phase of inflammatory arthritis. Ann Rheum Dis 2013;72(8):1420–4.
74. de Hair MJH, van de Sande MGH, Ramwadhdoebe TH, et al. Features of the synovium of individuals at risk of developing rheumatoid arthritis: implications for understanding preclinical rheumatoid arthritis. Arthritis Rheumatol 2014;66(3):513–22.
75. Das S, Padhan P. An overview of the extraarticular involvement in rheumatoid arthritis and its management. J Pharmacol Pharmacother 2017;8(3):81–6.
76. Deane KD, Norris JM, Holers VM. Preclinical rheumatoid arthritis: identification, evaluation, and future directions for investigation. Rheum Dis Clin North Am 2010;36(2):213–41.
77. Kurki P, Aho K, Palosuo T, et al. Immunopathology of rheumatoid arthritis. Anti-keratin antibodies precede the clinical disease. Arthritis Rheum 1992;35(8):914–7. Available at: http://www.ncbi.nlm.nih.gov/pubmed/1379430. Accessed April 19, 2018.
78. Nielen MMJ, van Schaardenburg D, Reesink HW, et al. Specific autoantibodies precede the symptoms of rheumatoid arthritis: a study of serial measurements in blood donors. Arthritis Rheum 2004;50(2):380–6.
79. van de Stadt LA, de Koning MHMT, van de Stadt RJ, et al. Development of the anti-citrullinated protein antibody repertoire prior to the onset of rheumatoid arthritis. Arthritis Rheum 2011;63(11):3226–33.
80. Shi J, Knevel R, Suwannalai P, et al. Autoantibodies recognizing carbamylated proteins are present in sera of patients with rheumatoid arthritis and predict joint damage. Proc Natl Acad Sci U S A 2011;108(42):17372–7.
81. Shi J, van Steenbergen HW, van Nies JAB, et al. The specificity of anti-carbamylated protein antibodies for rheumatoid arthritis in a setting of early arthritis. Arthritis Res Ther 2015;17:339.
82. Shi J, Van De Stadt LA, Levarht EWN, et al. Anti-carbamylated protein (anti-CarP) antibodies precede the onset of rheumatoid arthritis. Ann Rheum Dis 2014;73(4):780–3.
83. Thiele GM, Duryee MJ, Anderson DR, et al. Malondialdehyde-acetaldehyde adducts and anti-malondialdehyde-acetaldehyde antibodies in rheumatoid arthritis. Arthritis Rheumatol 2015;67(3):645–55.
84. Mikuls TR, Duryee MJ, Rahman R, et al. Enrichment of malondialdehyde-acetaldehyde antibody in the rheumatoid arthritis joint. Rheumatology 2017;56(10):1794–803.

85. Wigerblad G, Bas DB, Fernades-Cerqueira C, et al. Autoantibodies to citrullinated proteins induce joint pain independent of inflammation via a chemokine-dependent mechanism. Ann Rheum Dis 2016;75(4):730–8.

86. Harre U, Georgess D, Bang H, et al. Induction of osteoclastogenesis and bone loss by human autoantibodies against citrullinated vimentin. J Clin Invest 2012; 122(5):1791–802.

87. Scherer HU, van der Woude D, Ioan-Facsinay A, et al. Glycan profiling of anti-citrullinated protein antibodies isolated from human serum and synovial fluid. Arthritis Rheum 2010;62(6):1620–9.

88. Rombouts Y, Ewing E, van de Stadt LA, et al. Anti-citrullinated protein antibodies acquire a pro-inflammatory Fc glycosylation phenotype prior to the onset of rheumatoid arthritis. Ann Rheum Dis 2015;74(1):234–41.

89. Pfeifle R, Rothe T, Ipseiz N, et al. Regulation of autoantibody activity by the IL-23-TH17 axis determines the onset of autoimmune disease. Nat Immunol 2017; 18(1):104–13.

90. Molendijk M, Hazes JM, Lubberts E. From patients with arthralgia, pre-RA and recently diagnosed RA: what is the current status of understanding RA pathogenesis? RMD Open 2018;4(1):e000256.

91. Deane KD, O'Donnell CI, Hueber W, et al. The number of elevated cytokines and chemokines in preclinical seropositive rheumatoid arthritis predicts time to diagnosis in an age-dependent manner. Arthritis Rheum 2010;62(11):3161–72.

92. Kokkonen H, Söderström I, Rocklöv J, et al. Up-regulation of cytokines and chemokines predates the onset of rheumatoid arthritis. Arthritis Rheum 2010;62(2): 383–91.

93. Chalan P, Bijzet J, van den Berg A, et al. Analysis of serum immune markers in seropositive and seronegative rheumatoid arthritis and in high-risk seropositive arthralgia patients. Sci Rep 2016;6:26021.

94. Lee YC, Lu B, Boire G, et al. Incidence and predictors of secondary fibromyalgia in an early arthritis cohort. Ann Rheum Dis 2013;72(6):949–54.

95. Duffield SJ, Miller N, Zhao S, et al. Concomitant fibromyalgia complicating chronic inflammatory arthritis: a systematic review and meta-analysis. Rheumatology (Oxford) 2018;57(8):1453–60.

96. Bodnar RJ, Romero MT, Kramer E. Organismic variables and pain inhibition: roles of gender and aging. Brain Res Bull 1988. https://doi.org/10.1016/0361-9230(88)90032-9.

97. Romero MT, Kepler KL, Bodnar RJ. Gender determinants of opioid mediation of swim analgesia in rats. Pharmacol Biochem Behav 1988;29(4):705–9.

98. Fillingim RB, Maixner W. Gender differences in the responses to noxious stimuli. Pain Forum 1995;4(4):209–21. https://doi.org/10.1016/S1082-3174(11)80022-X.

99. Melchior M, Poisbeau P, Gaumond I, et al. Insights into the mechanisms and the emergence of sex-differences in pain. Neuroscience 2016;338:63–80.

100. Mogil JS. Qualitative sex differences in pain processing: emerging evidence of a biased literature. Nat Rev Neurosci 2020;21(7):353–65.

101. Rovner GS, Sunnerhagen KS, Björkdahl A, et al. Chronic pain and sex-differences; women accept and move, while men feel blue. PLoS One 2017; 12(4):1–12.

102. Fischer BD, Adeyemo A, O'Leary ME, et al. Animal models of rheumatoid pain: experimental systems and insights. Arthritis Res Ther 2017;19(1). https://doi.org/10.1186/s13075-017-1361-6.

103. Choudhary N, Bhatt LK, Prabhavalkar KS. Experimental animal models for rheumatoid arthritis. Immunopharmacol Immunotoxicol 2018;40(3):193–200.

104. Krock E, Jurczak A, Svensson CI. Pain pathogenesis in rheumatoid arthritis-what have we learned from animal models? Pain 2018;159(Suppl 1):S98–109.
105. Cook CD, Nickerson MD. Nociceptive sensitivity and opioid antinociception and antihyperalgesia in Freund's adjuvant-induced arthritic male and female rats. J Pharmacol Exp Ther 2005;313(1):449–59.
106. Chillingworth NL, Donaldson LF. Characterisation of a Freund's complete adjuvant-induced model of chronic arthritis in mice. J Neurosci Methods 2003;128(1–2):45–52. Available at: http://www.ncbi.nlm.nih.gov/pubmed/12948547. Accessed September 21, 2018.
107. Gauldie SD, McQueen DS, Clarke CJ, et al. A robust model of adjuvant-induced chronic unilateral arthritis in two mouse strains. J Neurosci Methods 2004;139(2):281–91.
108. Inglis JJ, Notley CA, Essex D, et al. Collagen-induced arthritis as a model of hyperalgesia: functional and cellular analysis of the analgesic actions of tumor necrosis factor blockade. Arthritis Rheum 2007;56(12):4015–23.
109. Kouskoff V, Korganow AS, Duchatelle V, et al. Organ-specific disease provoked by systemic autoimmunity. Cell 1996;87(5):811–22.
110. Christianson CA, Corr M, Firestein GS, et al. Characterization of the acute and persistent pain state present in K/BxN serum transfer arthritis. Pain 2010;151(2):394–403.
111. Ashraf S, Bouhana KS, Pheneger J, et al. Selective inhibition of tropomyosin-receptor-kinase A (TrkA) reduces pain and joint damage in two rat models of inflammatory arthritis. Arthritis Res Ther 2016;18(1):97.
112. Fernandez-Zafra T, Gao T, Jurczak A, et al. Exploring the transcriptome of resident spinal microglia after collagen antibody-induced arthritis. Pain 2019;160(1):224–36.
113. Woller SA, Ocheltree C, Wong SY, et al. Neuraxial TNF and IFN-beta co-modulate persistent allodynia in arthritic mice. Brain Behav Immun 2019;76:151–8.
114. Sun R-Q, Lawand NB, Willis WD. The role of calcitonin gene-related peptide (CGRP) in the generation and maintenance of mechanical allodynia and hyperalgesia in rats after intradermal injection of capsaicin. Pain 2003;104(1–2):201–8. Available at: http://www.ncbi.nlm.nih.gov/pubmed/12855330. Accessed August 17, 2018.
115. Vincent K, Tracey I. Hormones and their interaction with the pain experience. Rev Pain 2008. https://doi.org/10.1177/204946370800200206.
116. Tang MW, Garcia S, Gerlag DM, et al. Insight into the endocrine system and the immune system: a review of the inflammatory role of prolactin in rheumatoid arthritis and psoriatic arthritis. Front Immunol 2017;8(JUN):23.
117. Liu L, Jia J, Jiang M, et al. High susceptibility to collagen-induced arthritis in mice with progesterone receptors selectively inhibited in osteoprogenitor cells. Arthritis Res Ther 2020;22(1):1–12.
118. Bupp MRG, Jorgensen TN. Androgen-induced immunosuppression. Front Immunol 2018;9(APR):1. https://doi.org/10.3389/fimmu.2018.00794.
119. Yang DD, Krasnova A, Nead KT, et al. Androgen deprivation therapy and risk of rheumatoid arthritis in patients with localized prostate cancer. Ann Oncol 2018;29(2):386–91.
120. Baillargeon J, Al Snih S, Raji MA, et al. Hypogonadism and the risk of rheumatic autoimmune disease. Clin Rheumatol 2016;35(12):2983–7.
121. Keast JR, Gleeson RJ. Androgen receptor immunoreactivity is present in primary sensory neurons of male rats. Neuroreport 1998. https://doi.org/10.1097/00001756-199812210-00025.

122. Fanton LE, Macedo CG, Torres-Chávez KE, et al. Activational action of testosterone on androgen receptors protects males preventing temporomandibular joint pain. Pharmacol Biochem Behav 2017. https://doi.org/10.1016/j.pbb.2016.07.005.

123. Fischer L, Clemente JT, Tambeli CH. The protective role of testosterone in the development of temporomandibular joint pain. J Pain 2007. https://doi.org/10.1016/j.jpain.2006.12.007.

124. Lesnak JB, Inoue S, Lima L, et al. Testosterone protects against the development of widespread muscle pain in mice. Pain 2020. https://doi.org/10.1097/j.pain.0000000000001985.

125. Kato Y, Shigehara K, Kawaguchi S, et al. Efficacy of testosterone replacement therapy on pain in hypogonadal men with chronic pain syndrome: a subanalysis of a prospective randomised controlled study in Japan (EARTH study). Andrologia 2020. https://doi.org/10.1111/and.13768.

126. Gold MS, Flake NM. Inflammation-mediated hyperexcitability of sensory neurons. Neurosignals 2005;14(4):147–57.

127. Cho T, Chaban VV. Expression of P2X3 and TRPV1 receptors in primary sensory neurons from estrogen receptors-α and estrogen receptor-β knockout mice. Neuroreport 2012. https://doi.org/10.1097/WNR.0b013e328353fabc.

128. Taleghany N, Sarajari S, DonCarlos LL, et al. Differential expression of estrogen receptor alpha and beta in rat dorsal root ganglion neurons. J Neurosci Res 1999. https://doi.org/10.1002/(SICI)1097-4547(19990901)57:5<603::AID-JNR3>3.0.CO;2-R.

129. Lu Y, Jiang Q, Yu L, et al. 17β-estradiol rapidly attenuates P2X3 receptor-mediated peripheral pain signal transduction via ERα and GPR30. Endocrinology 2013. https://doi.org/10.1210/en.2012-2119.

130. Ma B, hua Yu L, Fan J, et al. Estrogen modulation of peripheral pain signal transduction: involvement of P2X3 receptors. Purinergic Signal 2011. https://doi.org/10.1007/s11302-010-9212-9.

131. Chaban V, Li J, McDonald JS, et al. Estradiol attenuates the adenosine triphosphate-induced increase of intracellular calcium through group II metabotropic glutamate receptors in rat dorsal root ganglion neurons. J Neurosci Res 2011. https://doi.org/10.1002/jnr.22718.

132. Cho T, Chaban VV. Interaction Between P2X3 and Oestrogen Receptor (ER)α/ERβ in ATP-Mediated Calcium Signalling In Mice Sensory Neurones. J Neuroendocrinol 2012;24(5):789–97. https://doi.org/10.1111/j.1365-2826.2011.02272.x.

133. Xu S, Cheng Y, Keast JR, et al. 17β-estradiol activates estrogen receptor β-signalling and inhibits transient receptor potential vanilloid receptor 1 activation by capsaicin in adult rat nociceptor neurons. Endocrinology 2008. https://doi.org/10.1210/en.2008-0278.

134. Nazarian A, Tenayuca JM, Almasarweh F, et al. Sex differences in formalin-evoked primary afferent release of substance P. Eur J Pain 2014. https://doi.org/10.1002/j.1532-2149.2013.00346.x.

135. Sohrabji F, Miranda RC, Toran-Allerand CD. Estrogen differentially regulates estrogen and nerve growth factor receptor mRNAs in adult sensory neurons. J Neurosci 1994. https://doi.org/10.1523/jneurosci.14-02-00459.1994.

136. Liuzzi FJ, Scoville SA, Bufton SM. Long-term estrogen replacement coordinately decreases trkA and β-PPT mRNA levels in dorsal root ganglion neurons. Exp Neurol 1999. https://doi.org/10.1006/exnr.1998.6999.

137. Lanlua P, Decorti F, Gangula PRR, et al. Female steroid hormones modulate receptors for nerve growth factor in rat dorsal root ganglia. Biol Reprod 2001. https://doi.org/10.1095/biolreprod64.1.331.

138. Garrett NE, Mapp PI, Cruwys SC, et al. Role of substance P in inflammatory arthritis. Ann Rheum Dis 1992. https://doi.org/10.1136/ard.51.8.1014.

139. Keeble JE, Brain SD. A role for substance P in arthritis? Neurosci Lett 2004. https://doi.org/10.1016/j.neulet.2003.12.020.

140. Denk F, Bennett DL, McMahon SB. Nerve growth factor and pain mechanisms. Annu Rev Neurosci April 2017. https://doi.org/10.1146/annurev-neuro-072116-031121.

141. Seidel MF, Herguijuela M, Forkert R, et al. Nerve growth factor in rheumatic diseases. Semin Arthritis Rheum 2010;40(2):109–26.

142. Yang Y, Ozawa H, Lu H, et al. Immunocytochemical analysis of sex differences in calcitonin gene- related peptide in the rat dorsal root ganglion, with special reference to estrogen and its receptor. Brain Res 1998. https://doi.org/10.1016/S0006-8993(98)00021-3.

143. Patil M, Belugin S, Mecklenburg J, et al. Prolactin regulates pain responses via a female-selective nociceptor-specific mechanism. iScience 2019;20:449–65.

144. Tang MW, Reedquist KA, Garcia S, et al. The prolactin receptor is expressed in rheumatoid arthritis and psoriatic arthritis synovial tissue and contributes to macrophage activation. Rheumatology (Oxford) 2016;55(12):2248–59.

145. Tavares-Ferreira D, Ray PR, Sankaranarayanan I, et al. Sex differences in nociceptor translatomes contribute to divergent prostaglandin signaling in male and female mice Short title: sex differences in mouse nociceptor translatomes. bioRxiv 2020. https://doi.org/10.1101/2020.07.31.231753.

146. Chillingworth NL, Morham SG, Donaldson LF. Sex differences in inflammation and inflammatory pain in cyclooxygenase-deficient mice. Am J Physiol Regul Integr Comp Physiol 2006;291(2):R327–34.

147. Dimitrijević M, Arsenović-Ranin N, Kosec D, et al. Sex differences in Tfh cell help to B cells contribute to sexual dimorphism in severity of rat collagen-induced arthritis. Sci Rep 2020;10(1):1–15.

148. Sorge RE, Mapplebeck JCS, Rosen S, et al. Different immune cells mediate mechanical pain hypersensitivity in male and female mice. Nat Neurosci 2015; 18(8):1081–3.

149. Sorge RE, LaCroix-Fralish ML, Tuttle AH, et al. Spinal cord toll-like receptor 4 mediates inflammatory and neuropathic hypersensitivity in male but not female mice. J Neurosci 2011;31(43):15450–4.

150. Zhang W j, Luo H l, Zhu Z m. The role of P2X4 receptors in chronic pain: a potential pharmacological target. Biomed Pharmacother 2020;129. https://doi.org/10.1016/j.biopha.2020.110447.

151. Halievski K, Ghazisaeidi S, Salter MW. Sex-dependent mechanisms of chronic pain: a focus on microglia and P2X4R. J Pharmacol Exp Ther 2020;120:265017.

152. Mapplebeck JCS, Dalgarno R, Tu YS, et al. Microglial P2X4R-evoked pain hypersensitivity is sexually dimorphic in rats. Pain 2018;159(9):1752–63.

153. Loyd DR, Murphy AZ. Androgen and estrogen (α) receptor localization on periaqueductal gray neurons projecting to the rostral ventromedial medulla in the male and female rat. J Chem Neuroanat 2008. https://doi.org/10.1016/j.jchemneu.2008.08.001.

154. Xiao X, Yang Y, Zhang Y, et al. Estrogen in the anterior cingulate cortex contributes to pain-related aversion. Cereb Cortex 2013. https://doi.org/10.1093/cercor/bhs201.

155. Traub RJ, Ji Y. Sex differences and hormonal modulation of deep tissue pain. Front Neuroendocrinol 2013;34(4):350–66.
156. Crofford LJ. Use of NSAIDs in treating patients with arthritis. Arthritis Res Ther 2013;15:S2. https://doi.org/10.1186/ar4174. Suppl 3(Suppl 3).
157. Christianson CA, Corr M, Yaksh TL, et al. K/BxN serum transfer arthritis as a model of inflammatory joint pain. Methods Mol Biol 2012;851:249–60.
158. Hurley RW, Adams MCB. Sex, gender, and pain: an overview of a complex field. Anesth Analg 2008;107(1):309–17.
159. Bartley EJ, Palit S. Gender and pain. Curr Anesthesiol Rep 2016;6(4):344–53.
160. Bartley EJ, Fillingim RB. Sex differences in pain: a brief review of clinical and experimental findings. Br J Anaesth 2013;111(1):52–8.
161. Berkley KJ, Zalcman SS, Simon VR. Sex and gender differences in pain and inflammation: a rapidly maturing field. Am J Physiol Regul Integr Comp Physiol 2006;291(2):241–4.
162. Greenspan JD, Craft RM, LeResche L, et al. Studying sex and gender differences in pain and analgesia: A consensus report. Pain 2007;132(SUPPL. 1): S26. https://doi.org/10.1016/j.pain.2007.10.014.
163. Kuba T, Quinones-Jenab V. The role of female gonadal hormones in behavioral sex differences in persistent and chronic pain: clinical versus preclinical studies. Brain Res Bull 2005;66(3):179–88.
164. Strassman AM, Mineta Y, Vos BP. Distribution of fos-like immunoreactivity in the medullary and upper cervical dorsal horn produced by stimulation of dural blood vessels in the rat. J Neurosci 1994;14(6):3725–35.

Cannabinoids and Pain
The Highs and Lows

Oliver Hulland, MD[a], Jessica Oswald, MD, MPH[b,c],*

KEYWORDS

- Marijuana • Cannabinoids • Chronic pain • CBD • THC

KEY POINTS

- Cannabinoids can be effective at treating some chronic pain.
- There is limited high-quality evidence regarding the use of cannabinoids in pain.
- Cannabinoids have opioid sparing properties and can be useful in treating pain.
- CBD may be useful in treating anxiety and improving sleep.

INTRODUCTION/BACKGROUND

Cannabis has been used medicinally for the treatment of pain for millennia, but its use in modern medicine has been encumbered by what can be described as an excess of public enthusiasm, a relative paucity of rigorous trials, and a minefield of politicization and regulatory challenges. Regardless of these challenges, the landscape of cannabis use is rapidly expanding, at least in the United States, with state legislatures adopting decriminalization and legalization above-and-beyond any purported therapeutic use within the medical setting. Because of this it is imperative that clinicians remain well versed in the literature to better explain and answer questions their patients might have about the relative benefits (and oft-ignored harms) of cannabis and its various pharmacologically active compounds. Specifically, we seek to separate the high from the hype with the hope that we can ground expectations regarding the use of cannabinoids in the treatment of pain.

RELEVANCE

Chronic pain is frequently stated as the primary reasons for the use of medical cannabis. In Colorado, 94% of marijuana identification holders indicated "severe pain" as a medical condition.[1] An earlier study evaluating patient characteristics in

[a] Department of Emergency Medicine, Yale-New Haven Hospital, Yale University, 464 Congress Avenue, New Haven, CT 06519, USA; [b] Center for Pain Medicine, Department of Anesthesiology, UC San Diego Health, La Jolla, CA, USA; [c] Department of Emergency Medicine, UC San Diego Health, La Jolla, CA, USA
* Corresponding author. UC San Diego Health Center for Pain Medicine, 9400 Campus Point Dr., La Jolla, CA 92037, USA.
E-mail address: jeoswald@health.ucsd.edu

Rheum Dis Clin N Am 47 (2021) 265–275
https://doi.org/10.1016/j.rdc.2020.12.005
0889-857X/21/© 2020 Elsevier Inc. All rights reserved.

2013 found that 87% of patients seeking medicinal marijuana cited using it for analgesia.[2] The demand for cannabis in the treatment of pain precedes formal approval by the United States Food and Drug Administration. Observational studies have shown that states with access to medical marijuana have had an associated reduction in the number of prescribed opioids and benzodiazepines.[3,4] With legalization of medical marijuana, patients are increasingly turning to marijuana as a potential treatment of their pain. The heterogeneity of cannabis compounds available on the marketplace ranging from synthetic and plant-based formulations, the varying routes of delivery (oral, smoke inhalation, vaping, topical), and the lack of standardization for dosing and quality increases the difficulty of researching cannabis and its cannabinoids. Most of the individual use is not representative of the cannabinoids studied in the currently available standardized trials.

CANNABINOIDS AND THEIR RECEPTORS

Cannabis is a genus of plants that includes *Cannabis sativa* that produce more than 500 compounds of which 107 are classified as phytocannabinoids.[5] Cannabinoids can be divided into 3 groups: phytocannabinoids, which are derived from the plant cannabis, endocannabinoids, which are endogenous compounds capable of interacting at cannabinoid receptors, and synthetic cannabinoids, which have been manufactured as pharmacologic products.[6] The primary psychoactive compound is the phytocannabinoid Δ9-tetrahydrocannabinol (Δ9-THC), which was isolated in 1967.[7] Outside of Δ9-THC, there are other important pharmacologically active phytocannabinoids including delta-8-tetrahydrocannabinol (Δ8-THC), cannabidiol (CBD), and cannabinol.[6] CBD is the second most abundant phytocannabinoid in cultivated marijuana and is minimally psychoactive but plays an important role in modulating the effects of other phytocannabinoids.[8] The primary endocannabinoids are anandamide (AEA) (ananda is Sanskrit for "bliss") and 2-arachidonoylglycerol (2-AG) [9](**Table 1**).

Cannabinoids function through binding to 2 receptors: the cannabinoid receptor type 1 (CB1) and CB2.[10] Both CB1 and CB2 function through the action of G protein–coupled receptors, which when agonized leads to the inhibition of adenylyl cyclase.[11] The 2 receptors, CB1 and CB2, and their associated ligands, anandamide and 2-arachidonoylglycerol, form the endocannabinoid system. CB1 receptors are commonly found throughout the central nervous system, whereas CB2 receptors are less widely distributed but can be found on immune and hematopoietic cells and play an important role in cytokine regulation.[12] CB1 receptors are most commonly presynaptic, and their stimulation via endocannabinoids leads to suppression of neuronal excitability, which inhibits neurotransmission.[13] This inhibition and the widespread distribution of CB1 receptors through the central nervous system suggests that the underlying function of the endocannabinoid system may be to suppress excessive neuronal activity through modulation of inhibitory and excitatory

| Table 1 | | |
| Cannabinoids and their receptors | | |
Endocannabinoids	Phytocannabinoids	Synthetic Cannabinoids
Anandamide (AEA)	Tetrahydrocannibinol (THC)	Dronabinol
2-Arachidonylglycerol (2-AG)	Cannabidiol (CBD)	Nabilone
	Cannabichromene (CBC)	Lenabasum
	Cannabigerol (CBG)	

neurotransmitters, including acetylcholine, noradrenaline, dopamine, 5-hydroxytryptamine, g-aminobutyric acid, glutamate, D-aspartate, and cholecystokinin.[8,11] There is evidence that phytocannabinoids such as Δ9-THC may directly affect other receptors, with several studies finding it functions as a partial agonist on mu-opioid receptors.[14–16] In addition, cannabinoids acting at CB2 receptors have been shown to directly increase release of endogenous opioids.[17] This likely accounts, at least in part, for the opioid-sparing effect seen with coadministration of cannabinoids.[18]

In contrast to the agonism that Δ9-THC has on CB1 and CB2, the role of CBD is distinctly different. Notably, CBD has low affinity for CB1 and CB2 but has demonstrated activity as an antagonist and "inverse agonist" with meaningful downregulation of CB2, which has been shown to contribute to an antiinflammatory effect by modulating cytokine release.[8,19] CBD may indirectly affect pain via antiinflammatory and anxiolytic properties. One potential mechanism of action is the purported CBD inhibition of fatty acid amide hydrolase, the enzyme hydrolyzing the endocannabinoid N-arachidonoylethanolamine (AEA). Boosting AEA levels may be a therapeutic strategy, as evidenced in animal studies and in one human study of CBD for psychosis in patients with schizophrenia.[20,21]

Δ9-THC has antinociceptive effects through agonism of CB1 and CB2 cannabinoid receptors, located centrally and peripherally.[22,23] CB2 inhibits the inflammatory pain response, indirectly activates opioid receptors via primary afferent pathways, and is upregulated in neuropathic pain at the dorsal root ganglia.[17,24] THC has been shown to be an effective analgesic and has antinociceptive synergy when combined with opioids, providing opioid-sparing effects.[18,25–28] The analgesic mechanisms of CBD remain poorly understood and may be occurring at noncannabinoid receptors.[29]

PHARMACOLOGY OF CANNABINOIDS

The pharmacokinetics of cannabinoids depends on formulation and method of administration. Inhalation is equivalent to intravenous administration in terms of time to peak plasma concentration of both THC and CBD with a time to peak concentration ranging between 3 and 10 minutes.[30] When inhaled, THC has a bioavailability of 10% to 35% (the wide range is secondary to the variability related to inhalation technique and the device), and CBD has a similar bioavailability of 31%.[30] This is in contrast with oral absorption wherein there is first-pass metabolism of both THC and CBD with a bioavailability of about 6% and delayed peak plasma concentration of 60 to 120 minutes.[30,31] The substantial delays in oral administration account for many of the difficulties in self-titration with edible THC products. Oromucosal administration avoids these effects and has similar characteristics to inhalation with some delay likely secondary to oral ingestion. The metabolism of THC is hepatic via cytochrome p450 isozymes CYP2C9, CYP2C19, and CYP3A4; similarly, CBD is hepatically metabolized via CYP2C19 and CYP3A4, and both are excreted in the urine and feces.[30] Notably, THC is highly lipophilic and is able to cross the placenta and is excreted into breast milk.[32]

PHARMACOLOGIC OR MEDICAL TREATMENT OPTIONS

In addition to herbal marijuana, there are several pharmaceutical preparations containing cannabinoids: nabiximols (Sativex), dronabinol (Marinol), nabilone (Cesamet), and plant-derived CBD (Epidiolex).

Herbal marijuana is a heterogenous source of cannabinoids, posing a challenge in evaluating its clinical efficacy. It is primarily smoked and inhaled but can also be consumed orally, vaporized, or applied topically. The concentration of Δ9-THC and CBD varies substantially between plant strains, growing environment, and product preparation. A recent evaluation of cannabis grown and sold at dispensaries in the United States found the average Δ9-THC concentration to be greater than 24% with a corresponding decrease in CBD concentration as Δ9-THC increased.[33] A recent study in JAMA evaluating labeling of cannabinoid containing products at dispensaries found that approximately 17% were accurately labeled with regard to THC content; of the products evaluated there was a mean THC:CBD ratio of 36:1, a THC ratio that is higher than what has been studied previously.[34] These higher concentrations of Δ9-THC are distinct when compared with the currently available literature, demonstrating efficacy in the treatment of neuropathic pain with concentrations of Δ9-THC ranging from 5% to 10%.[25,35,36] As the Δ9-THC content increases the rate of adverse side effects increase, with some studies demonstrating a dose-dependent *hyperalgesic effect*.[37,38] Inhaled medical cannabis containing both Δ9-THC and CBD has been shown to decrease treatment refractory neuropathic pain in a dose-responsive manner.[25,37,38]

Nabiximols (Sativex) is a whole plant–derived oromucosal formulation of a 1:1 ratio of THC:CBD approved in Canada and several European countries for the treatment multiple sclerosis (MS) related.[39] Its formulation allows for a consistent dose of 2.7 mg of THC and 2.5 mg of CBD per spray, with rapid onset of effects occurring within 15 to 40 minutes allowing for titration to effect. The combination of CBD and THC seems to balance the partial agonism of CB1 and CB2 with an antagonistic effect from CBD, which serves to amplify some of the beneficial effects while ameliorating many of the adverse effects with evidence suggesting it also reduces the risk of dependence.[40] Sativex has been well studied in MS, demonstrating a reduction in MS-related spasticity, MS-related pain, and improved sleep.[41–43] Outside of MS, there have been 2 trials involving neuropathic pain, one involving brachial plexus avulsion and another involving unilateral neuropathic pain, where Sativex was found to substantially reduce pain and improve quality of sleep.[44,45] It is currently not approved by Food and Drug Administration (FDA) in the United States but is undergoing phase III trials for it therapeutic efficacy in cancer-related pain.

Dronabinol (Marinol) is a synthetic form of delta-9-THC that is FDA approved for the treatment of nausea associated with chemotherapy and used as an appetite stimulant for human immunodeficiency virus (HIV)-related wasting syndrome.[8] Dronabinol has been studied as an adjuvant to opioid therapy in the treatment of chronic pain, with significant increase in pain relief and satisfaction.[46] Nabilone is another synthetic analogue of THC, which is more potent than dronabinol. It has been shown to have a modest effect on reduction of pain scores, with improvement of secondary outcomes including sleep and anxiety.[47] Both are currently FDA approved in the United States to treat chemotherapy-associated nausea and vomiting.

COMPLICATIONS

One of the greatest challenges facing the evaluation and use of cannabinoids in the treatment of pain is the associated side effects and potential for abuse and dependence. These effects are variable and dose dependent. THC can cause euphoria, dizziness, anxiety, tachycardia, dry mouth, decreased body temperature, hypotension, paranoia, somnolence, and impaired concentration and memory.[48] There is evidence that heavy use of cannabis increases the risk of psychosis and schizophrenia.[49,50] CBD, in comparison, has not been shown to have any significant side effects in humans either at high doses or with chronic use when studied in isolation.[51] When used in conjunction with THC, CBD has been shown to ameliorate the psychoactive properties of THC.[19,40,51] The frequency with which adverse effects occur is very high, with a recent systematic review and meta-analysis in 2018 demonstrating that the OR of adverse effects was 2.33 (1.88–2.89) when compared with placebo with thought disturbance (odds ratio [OR] 7.35), dizziness (OR 5.52), and confusion listed as the most common adverse events.[52] It should be noted that most of the adverse effects are nonserious and that there are no substantiated reports of death from overdose of either THC or CBD.[51,53,54] In a 1-year prospective cohort trial titled Cannabis for the Management of Pain: Assessment of Safety Study (COMPASS) medical cannabis users had no increased risk of serious adverse events when compared with placebo but did have a significant increase in nonserious adverse events.[55] An additional complication arising from marijuana use is dependence, with up to 8% of users of nonmedical cannabis developing dependence; however, this subject is not well studied within medical cannabis users.[56]

THE EVIDENCE FOR CANNABINOIDS AND PAIN

There are few high-quality randomized control trials evaluating the use of cannabinoids as they relate to pain, inflammation, sleep, and anxiety. Those that do exist predominantly address neuropathic pain, with relatively fewer studies addressing acute pain, inflammatory pain, and cancer pain. To date, the most comprehensive systematic review evaluating the medical use of cannabinoids was published by Whiting and colleagues[57] in 2015. The review included 28 randomized controlled trials (RCT) in patients with chronic pain including 2454 participants and found that the average number of patients who reported a reduction of neuropathic or cancer pain by at least 30% was greater with cannabinoids than with placebo with an OR of 1.4. Based on this systematic review, including a few smaller more recent trials, the National Academies of Sciences, Engineering and Medicine published a consensus study stating there was substantial evidence to support the use of cannabinoids in the treatment of chronic pain.[50]

In contrast to Whiting and colleagues, a systematic review by Stockings and colleagues in 2018 focused specifically on the use of cannabinoids in the treatment of chronic noncancer pain broadened the review criteria to include 47 RCTs and 57 observational trials including 9958 participants. The results found that 29% of participants taking cannabinoids compared with 25.9% using placebo reported a 30% reduction in pain with a number needed to treat of 24 and a number needed to harm of 6.[52] Their findings report there is no high-quality evidence to support the use of cannabinoids in chronic noncancer pain. A more focused systematic review in 2016 of RCTs evaluating the use of cannabinoids in the treatment of chronic pain associated with rheumatic disease including fibromyalgia, chronic spinal pain, and rheumatoid arthritis similarly found that there was insufficient evidence to support their use.[58]

Less is known about CBD and how it affects pain and anxiety. A preliminary crossover study of 24 patients reported that CBD was effective in treating neuropathic pain. However, this was a cannabis medical extract (called "CBD-rich"); it is possible the therapeutic benefit was from other natural phytocannabinoids.[59] There have only been 2 other prospective trials of CBD for pain in humans, with small data sets and incomplete analyses.[60,61] CBD has been shown to reduce anxiety in social settings, and this anxiolytic effect may indirectly account for improvement in pain.[62,63] Approximately 50% of patients with chronic pain have anxiety-potentiated, pain-related disability scores.[64] CBD has been shown to have a dose-dependent impact on increasing overall length of sleep, which may benefit patients with pain-related insomnia.[65]

The evidence regarding the use of cannabinoids in chronic pain is mixed and of low quality. Although some research suggests cannabinoids are helpful in cancer and neuropathic pain, further research is needed to understand and draw conclusions if they are effective in nociceptive and other inflammatory pain syndromes.

NEW DEVELOPMENTS

Research involving cannabis has, by and large, focused on delta-9-THC at the expense of the minimally psychoactive and less well-understood CBD. Recently, efforts have been made to better elucidate the mechanism of CBD and evaluate its utility apart from THC in a wide variety of painful conditions, which has been helped by the 2018 FDA approval of Epidiolex as a treatment of intractable epilepsy and Lennox-Gastaut seizures and a rescheduling of medicinal CBD as a schedule V substance.[66,67]

There is emerging interest in the topical application of CBD in the form of oils and emollients with an associated proliferation of untested products available on the market. A recent trial involving inflammatory skin diseases demonstrated improvement of skin inflammation and scar formation after topical application of CBD.[68] Topical CBD has also been shown to reduce neuropathy-associated pain scores in podiatric patients with peripheral neuropathy in their feet.[69]

One of the primary attributes of CBD is its lack of agonism at CB1, which avoids many of the psychoactive, and therefore adoption-limiting, adverse effects of THC. There is increasing interest in developing synthetic cannabinoids that minimize CB1 agonism.[70] One recent candidate is lenabasum, a synthetic analogue of THC-8 with minimal CB1 agonism and increased selectivity for the CB2 receptor thought to have potent antiinflammatory properties.[71–73] A recent phase II clinical trial of lenabasum as a treatment of systemic sclerosis as well as dermatomyositis was completed and found to have no significant adverse effects, with significant reduction in disease severity and pain.[74,75]

SUMMARY AND FUTURE DIRECTIONS

The heterogeneity of product, different routes of delivery, and wide array of phytocannabinoids make cannabinoids difficult to study. The patchy regulatory framework around cannabis has created a poorly regulated marketplace with little standardization in terms of active ingredients. However, there seems to be a consistent signal demonstrating opioid-sparing effects and modest efficacy regarding the use of cannabinoids in the treatment of neuropathic and cancer-related pain. Early research demonstrates CBD may improve sleep quality and anxiety. More research and RCTs are needed to evaluate the safety and efficacy of cannabinoids as they relate to anxiety, sleep, and pain.

CLINICS CARE POINTS

- Cannabinoids can be useful in treating pain and have been shown to have opioid-sparing properties.
- CBD is not psychoactive and may be useful in treating pain-associated conditions including sleep quality and anxiety.
- Preferentially selecting cannabis products containing a lower THC:CBD ratio reduces undesirable psychoactive side effects and likely improves its efficacy in treating chronic pain.

DISCLOSURE

The authors have nothing to disclose.

REFERENCES

1. Light MK, Orens A, Lewandowski B, et al. Market size and demand for marijuana in Colorado. Denver, CO: Marijuana Policy Group; 2015.
2. Ilgen MA, Bohnert K, Kleinberg F, et al. Characteristics of adults seeking medical marijuana certification. Drug Alcohol Depend 2013;132(3):654–9.
3. Bradford AC, Bradford WD. Medical marijuana laws reduce prescription medication use in medicare part D. Health Aff 2016;35(7):1230–6.
4. Boehnke KF, Scott JR, Litinas E, et al. Pills to pot: observational analyses of cannabis substitution among medical cannabis users with chronic pain. J Pain 2019;20(7):830–41.
5. Amin MR, Ali DW. Pharmacology of medical cannabis. Adv Exp Med Biol 2019; 1162:151–65.
6. Ben Amar M. Cannabinoids in medicine: a review of their therapeutic potential. J Ethnopharmacol 2006;105(1–2):1–25.
7. Gaoni Y, Mechoulam R. Isolation, structure, and partial synthesis of an active constituent of hashish. J Am Chem Soc 1964;86(8):1646–7.
8. Pertwee RG. The diverse CB1 and CB2 receptor pharmacology of three plant cannabinoids: delta9-tetrahydrocannabinol, cannabidiol and delta9-tetrahydrocannabivarin. Br J Pharmacol 2008;153(2):199–215.
9. Castillo PE, Younts TJ, Chávez AE, et al. Endocannabinoid signaling and synaptic function. Neuron 2012;76(1):70–81.
10. Mackie K. Cannabinoid receptors: where they are and what they do. J Neuroendocrinol 2008;20(Suppl 1):10–4.
11. Howlett AC, Barth F, Bonner TI, et al. International Union of Pharmacology. XXVII. Classification of cannabinoid receptors. Pharmacol Rev 2002;54(2):161–202.
12. Hu SS-J, Mackie K. Distribution of the Endocannabinoid System in the Central Nervous System. Handb Exp Pharmacol 2015;231:59–93.
13. Freund TF, Katona I, Piomelli D. Role of endogenous cannabinoids in synaptic signaling. Physiol Rev 2003;83(3):1017–66.
14. Schoffelmeer AN, Hogenboom F, Wardeh G, et al. Interactions between CB1 cannabinoid and mu opioid receptors mediating inhibition of neurotransmitter release in rat nucleus accumbens core. Neuropharmacology 2006;51(4):773–81.
15. Cichewicz DL, Martin ZL, Smith FL, et al. Enhancement mu opioid antinociception by oral delta9-tetrahydrocannabinol: dose-response analysis and receptor identification. J Pharmacol Exp Ther 1999;289(2):859–67.
16. Christie MJ. Opioid and cannabinoid receptors: friends with benefits or just close friends? Br J Pharmacol 2006;148(4):385–6.
17. Ibrahim MM, Porreca F, Lai J, et al. CB2 cannabinoid receptor activation produces antinociception by stimulating peripheral release of endogenous opioids. Proc Natl Acad Sci U S A 2005;102(8):3093–8.
18. Nielsen S, Sabioni P, Trigo JM, et al. Opioid-sparing effect of cannabinoids: a systematic review and meta-analysis. Neuropsychopharmacology 2017;42(9):1752–65.
19. Laprairie RB, Bagher AM, Kelly ME, et al. Cannabidiol is a negative allosteric modulator of the cannabinoid CB1 receptor. Br J Pharmacol 2015;172(20):4790–805.

20. Leweke FM, Piomelli D, Pahlisch F, et al. Cannabidiol enhances anandamide signaling and alleviates psychotic symptoms of schizophrenia. Transl Psychiatry 2012;2:e94.

21. Caprioli A, Coccurello R, Rapino C, et al. The novel reversible fatty acid amide hydrolase inhibitor ST4070 increases endocannabinoid brain levels and counteracts neuropathic pain in different animal models. J Pharmacol Exp Ther 2012; 342(1):188–95.

22. Elikottil J, Gupta P, Gupta K. The analgesic potential of cannabinoids. J Opioid Manag 2009;5(6):341–57.

23. Marsicano G, Lutz B. Expression of the cannabinoid receptor CB1 in distinct neuronal subpopulations in the adult mouse forebrain. Eur J Neurosci 1999; 11(12):4213–25.

24. Zhang J, Hoffert C, Vu HK, et al. Induction of CB2 receptor expression in the rat spinal cord of neuropathic but not inflammatory chronic pain models. Eur J Neurosci 2003;17(12):2750–4.

25. Wallace MS, Marcotte TD, Umlauf A, et al. Efficacy of Inhaled Cannabis on Painful Diabetic Neuropathy. J Pain 2015;16(7):616–27.

26. Naef M, Curatolo M, Petersen-Felix S, et al. The analgesic effect of oral delta-9-tetrahydrocannabinol (THC), morphine, and a THC-morphine combination in healthy subjects under experimental pain conditions. Pain 2003;105(1–2):79–88.

27. Cichewicz DL, McCarthy EA. Antinociceptive synergy between delta(9)-tetrahydrocannabinol and opioids after oral administration. J Pharmacol Exp Ther 2003;304(3):1010–5.

28. Hickernell TR. Department of Orthopedic Surgery, Center for Hip, Knee Replacement, NewYork-Presbyterian Hospital Columbia University Medical Center New York New York, et al. Should cannabinoids be added to multimodal pain regimens after total hip and knee arthroplasty? J Arthroplasty 2020;33(12):3637–41.

29. Xiong W, Cui T, Cheng K, et al. Cannabinoids suppress inflammatory and neuropathic pain by targeting alpha3 glycine receptors. J Exp Med 2012;209(6): 1121–34.

30. Lucas CJ, Galettis P, Schneider J. The pharmacokinetics and the pharmacodynamics of cannabinoids. Br J Clin Pharmacol 2018;84(11):2477–82.

31. Agurell S, Halldin M, Lindgren JE, et al. Pharmacokinetics and metabolism of delta 1-tetrahydrocannabinol and other cannabinoids with emphasis on man. Pharmacol Rev 1986;38(1):21–43.

32. Perez-Reyes M, Wall ME. Presence of delta9-tetrahydrocannabinol in human milk. N Engl J Med 1982;307(13):819–20.

33. Cash MC, Cunnane K, Fan C, et al. Mapping cannabis potency in medical and recreational programs in the United States. PLoS One 2020;15(3):e0230167.

34. Bonn-Miller MO, Loflin MJE, Thomas BF, et al. Labeling accuracy of cannabidiol extracts sold online. JAMA 2017;318(17):1708–9.

35. Wilsey B, Marcotte T, Deutsch R, et al. Low-dose vaporized cannabis significantly improves neuropathic pain. J Pain 2013;14(2):136–48.

36. Abrams DI, Jay CA, Shade SB, et al. Cannabis in painful HIV-associated sensory neuropathy: a randomized placebo-controlled trial. Neurology 2007;68(7): 515–21.

37. Andreae MH, Carter GM, Shaparin N, et al. Inhaled cannabis for chronic neuropathic pain: a meta-analysis of individual patient data. J Pain 2015;16(12): 1221–32.

38. Wallace M, Schulteis G, Atkinson JH, et al. Dose-dependent effects of smoked cannabis on capsaicin-induced pain and hyperalgesia in healthy volunteers. Anesthesiology 2007;107(5):785–96.

39. Vermersch P, Trojano M. Tetrahydrocannabinol:Cannabidiol Oromucosal Spray for Multiple Sclerosis-Related Resistant Spasticity in Daily Practice. Eur Neurol 2016;76(5–6):216–26.

40. Russo E, Guy GW. A tale of two cannabinoids: the therapeutic rationale for combining tetrahydrocannabinol and cannabidiol. Med Hypotheses 2006;66(2): 234–46.

41. Nielsen S, Germanos R, Weier M, et al. The use of cannabis and cannabinoids in treating symptoms of multiple sclerosis: a systematic review of reviews. Curr Neurol Neurosci Rep 2018;18(2):8.

42. Rice J, Cameron M. Cannabinoids for Treatment of MS Symptoms: State of the Evidence. Curr Neurol Neurosci Rep 2018;18(8):50.

43. Ferrè L, Nuara A, Pavan G, et al. Efficacy and safety of nabiximols (Sativex(®)) on multiple sclerosis spasticity in a real-life Italian monocentric study. Neurol Sci 2016;37(2):235–42.

44. Nurmikko TJ, Serpell MG, Hoggart B, et al. Sativex successfully treats neuropathic pain characterised by allodynia: a randomised, double-blind, placebo-controlled clinical trial. Pain 2007;133(1–3):210–20.

45. Berman JS, Symonds C, Birch R. Efficacy of two cannabis based medicinal extracts for relief of central neuropathic pain from brachial plexus avulsion: results of a randomised controlled trial. Pain 2004;112(3):299–306.

46. Narang S, Gibson D, Wasan AD, et al. Efficacy of dronabinol as an adjuvant treatment for chronic pain patients on opioid therapy. J Pain 2008;9(3):254–64.

47. Tsang CC, Giudice MG. Nabilone for the management of pain. Pharmacotherapy 2016;36(3):273–86.

48. Borgelt LM, Franson KL, Nussbaum AM, et al. The pharmacologic and clinical effects of medical cannabis. Pharmacotherapy 2013;33(2):195–209.

49. Marconi A, Di Forti M, Lewis CM, et al. Meta-analysis of the association between the level of cannabis use and risk of psychosis. Schizophr Bull 2016;42(5): 1262–9.

50. National Academies of Sciences, Engineering, and Medicine, Health and Medicine Division, Board on Population Health and Public Health Practice, Committee on the Health Effects of Marijuana: An Evidence Review and Research Agenda. The health effects of cannabis and cannabinoids: the current state of evidence and recommendations for research. Washington DC: National Academies Press (US); 2017.

51. Bergamaschi MM, Queiroz RH, Zuardi AW, et al. Safety and side effects of cannabidiol, a Cannabis sativa constituent. Curr Drug Saf 2011;6(4):237–49.

52. Stockings E, Campbell G, Hall WD, et al. Cannabis and cannabinoids for the treatment of people with chronic noncancer pain conditions: a systematic review and meta-analysis of controlled and observational studies. Pain 2018;159(10): 1932–54.

53. Iffland K, Grotenhermen F. An Update on Safety and Side Effects of Cannabidiol: A Review of Clinical Data and Relevant Animal Studies. Cannabis Cannabinoid Res 2017;2(1):139–54.

54. Grotenhermen F. Pharmacokinetics and pharmacodynamics of cannabinoids. Clin Pharmacokinet 2003;42(4):327–60.

55. Ware MA, Wang T, Shapiro S, et al, COMPASS study team. Cannabis for the management of pain: assessment of safety study (COMPASS). J Pain 2015;16(12): 1233–42.
56. Lopez-Quintero C, de los Cobos JP, Hasin DS, et al. Probability and predictors of transition from first use to dependence on nicotine, alcohol, cannabis, and cocaine: Results of the National Epidemiologic Survey on Alcohol and Related Conditions (NESARC). Drug Alcohol Depend 2011;115(1):120–30.
57. Whiting PF, Wolff RF, Deshpande S, et al. Cannabinoids for Medical Use: A Systematic Review and Meta-analysis. JAMA 2015;313(24):2456–73.
58. Fitzcharles MA, Baerwald C, Ablin J, Häuser W. . Efficacy, tolerability and safety of cannabinoids in chronic pain associated with rheumatic diseases (fibromyalgia syndrome, back pain, osteoarthritis .... Der Schmerz. 2016. Available at: https://link.springer.com/content/pdf/10.1007/s00482-015-0084-3.pdf. Accessed September 16th, 2020.
59. Wade DT, Robson P, House H, et al. A preliminary controlled study to determine whether whole-plant cannabis extracts can improve intractable neurogenic symptoms. Clin Rehabil 2003;17(1):21–9.
60. Palmieri B, Laurino C, Vadala M. Short-Term Efficacy of CBD-enriched hemp oil in girls with dysautonomic syndrome after human papillomavirus vaccination. Isr Med Assoc J 2017;19(2):79–84.
61. Cunetti L, Manzo L, Peyraube R, et al. Chronic pain treatment with cannabidiol in kidney transplant patients in uruguay. Transpl Proc 2018;50(2):461–4.
62. Crippa JAS, Derenusson GN, Ferrari TB, et al. Neural basis of anxiolytic effects of cannabidiol (CBD) in generalized social anxiety disorder: a preliminary report. J Psychopharmacol 2011;25(1):121–30.
63. Bergamaschi MM, Queiroz RH, Chagas MH, et al. Cannabidiol reduces the anxiety induced by simulated public speaking in treatment-naive social phobia patients. Neuropsychopharmacology 2011;36(6):1219–26.
64. Lerman SF, Rudich Z, Brill S, et al. Longitudinal associations between depression, anxiety, pain, and pain-related disability in chronic pain patients. Psychosom Med 2015;77(3):333–41.
65. Nicholson AN, Turner C, Stone BM, et al. Effect of Delta-9-tetrahydrocannabinol and cannabidiol on nocturnal sleep and early-morning behavior in young adults. J Clin Psychopharmacol 2004;24(3):305–13.
66. Corroon J, Kight R. Regulatory status of cannabidiol in the united states: a perspective. Cannabis Cannabinoid Res 2018;3(1):190–4.
67. Drug Enforcement Administration. Schedules of controlled substances: placement in Schedule V of Certain FDA-approved drugs containing cannabidiol; corresponding change to permit requirements. Fed Regist 2018;83:48950–3.
68. Palmieri B, Laurino C, Vadalà M. A therapeutic effect of cbd-enriched ointment in inflammatory skin diseases and cutaneous scars. Clin Ter 2019;170(2):e93–9.
69. Xu DH, Cullen* BD, Tang M, et al. The effectiveness of topical cannabidiol oil in symptomatic relief of peripheral neuropathy of the lower extremities. Curr Pharm Biotechnol 2020;21(5):390–402.
70. Stasiulewicz A, Znajdek K, Grudzień M, et al. A guide to targeting the endocannabinoid system in drug design. Int J Mol Sci 2020;21(8). https://doi.org/10.3390/ijms21082778.
71. Motwani MP, Bennett F, Norris PC, et al. Potent anti-inflammatory and pro-resolving effects of anabasum in a human model of self-resolving acute inflammation. Clin Pharmacol Ther 2018;104(4):675–86.

72. Tepper MA, Zurier RB, Burstein SH. Ultrapure ajulemic acid has improved CB2 selectivity with reduced CB1 activity. Bioorg Med Chem 2014;22(13):3245–51.

73. Burstein SH. Ajulemic acid: potential treatment for chronic inflammation. Pharmacol Res Perspect 2018;6(2):e00394.

74. Spiera R, Hummers L, Chung L, et al. Safety and efficacy of lenabasum in a phase 2 randomized, placebo-controlled trial in adults with systemic sclerosis. Arthritis Rheumatol 2020;72(8):1350–60. Available at: https://onlinelibrary.wiley.com/doi/abs/10.1002/art.41294.

75. Werth VP, Hejazi E, Pena SM, et al. FRI0470 A phase 2 study of safety and efficacy of lenabasum (JBT-101), a cannabinoid receptor type 2 agonist, in refractory skin-predominant dermatomyositis. Ann Rheum Dis 2018;77(Suppl 2):763–4.

Nonpharmacologic Pain Management in Inflammatory Arthritis

Alexander Martin, MD[a], Ratnesh Chopra, MD[a],*,
Perry M. Nicassio, PhD[b]

KEYWORDS

- Pain • Inflammatory • Arthritis • Nonpharmacologic • Spondyloarthritis
- Rheumatoid • Psoriatic • Ankylosing

KEY POINTS

- An integrative approach to pain in inflammatory arthritis improves pain outcomes for patients.
- Many non-pharmacologic modalities of pain management have an evidence base for their efficacy in inflammatory arthritis.
- Maintenance of non-pharmacologic modalities of pain management is often required for ongoing benefit.

BACKGROUND

Inflammatory arthritis represents a group of chronic conditions comprised of rheumatoid arthritis (RA) and spondyloarthritides (SpA) that together affect approximately 3% of the global population.[1] Uncontrolled symptoms of inflammatory arthritis reduce quality of life in multiple domains; chief among these, in prevalence and degree of effect, is pain.[2-7] Pharmacologic therapies with antirheumatic drugs form a cornerstone of effective treatment of these diseases with a goal of controlling symptoms and arresting irreversible skeletal changes, but pain can prove refractory to antirheumatic drug titration.[5,8-10] Most measures of disease activity in inflammatory arthritis reflect a patients' experience of their disease by incorporating a subjective rating of disease activity, which is strongly influenced by pain.[5] Treating residual chronic pain pharmacologically introduces avoidable risk of potentially serious side effects, begging the question of what nonpharmacologic modalities are best suited to address the symptoms of pain and disability that patients with inflammatory arthritis experience.[11]

[a] Division of Rheumatology, UMass Medical School, 119 Belmont Street, Worcester, MA 01605, USA; [b] Department of Psychiatry, UCLA, 760 Westwood Plaza, C9-402, Los Angeles, CA 90095, USA
* Corresponding author.
E-mail address: Ratnesh.Chopra@umassmemorial.org

Rheum Dis Clin N Am 47 (2021) 277–295
https://doi.org/10.1016/j.rdc.2020.12.009
0889-857X/21/© 2020 Elsevier Inc. All rights reserved.

The experience of pain in chronic disease is a complex process that is influenced by multiple domains of health.[12] The biopsychosocial model of health provides a framework through which to address those domains that contribute to pain in inflammatory arthritis.[12] This framework seeks to address the subjective experience of objective biologic events through biologic, psychological, and social lenses.[12] Antirheumatic drugs target the biologic etiologies of lived disease activity, but psychological and social domains require interventions beyond pharmacologic treatment to address appropriately.

SELF-EFFICACY: THE FOUNDATIONAL PRINCIPLE

Self-efficacy is a mutable, domain-specific belief held by patients in their ability to effectively achieve goals by performing specific behaviors.[13–15] This belief has influences on patients' behaviors, thought patterns, and emotional reactions.[16] A higher degree of perceived self-efficacy has been shown to be correlated with improvements in many factors of health-related quality-of-life measures including pain intensity, coping capacity, response, and adherence to treatment.[17–22] Reduced levels of perceived affect and control (contributors to self-efficacy) have been associated with loss- and potential reversal-of-effect of nonpharmacologic pain treatments.[23] Bandura[13] proposed that self-efficacy is built on four major sources of information: (1) performance accomplishments, (2) vicarious experience, (3) verbal persuasion, and (4) physiologic states. These foundational sources of information can be fostered to improve self-efficacy, with ripple effects to improve perceived pain, disability, and ability to engage with other nonpharmacologic treatments.[13,24]

Self-efficacy's multifactorial cause offers choice in approaching its development. Implementation of a system of patient-centered communication has been shown to significantly improve self-efficacy.[25] Group activities, such as structured walking programs in patients with arthritis, promote self-efficacy via vicarious experience and personal achievement, demonstrating self-efficacy benefit at 6 weeks compared with similar, self-directed programs.[26,27]

Some psychosocial therapies targeted at pain management have shown correlation with benefit to self-efficacy, although teasing out the cause-effect relationship in this case is particularly difficult given the feedback loop between effective effortful therapies and self-efficacy.[14,28] Development of self-efficacy via personal experience has the added benefit of generalizability to other situations previously compromised by preoccupation with personal inadequacies.[13] Both cognitive behavioral therapy (CBT) and mindfulness-based interventions (MBI) have shown significant benefit in this domain.[14]

COGNITIVE BEHAVIORAL THERAPY

CBT is a form of therapy that seeks to modify thoughts and behaviors to give patients a sense of control over their emotions and symptoms.[29] It typically encompasses a series of individual or group sessions in which coping skills, such as relaxation, imagery, activity pacing, cognitive restructuring, and goal setting, are taught so that they can be used in the clinical and home settings.[12,30]

Rheumatoid Arthritis

CBT is among the most well-studied psychological pain interventions and demonstrates more robust evidence for pain control than MBIs or patient education (PE).[28] CBT has shown significant improvement in pain and self-efficacy in patients with RA.[28,31–33] Systematic review has found this effect only in therapy plans that include 6 or more weeks of CBT with conflicting evidence of persistent benefit at long-term follow-up of 6 to 12 months.[33,34] Prolonging the effects of CBT may be possible through "booster" sessions months after completing initial therapy.[30,35]

Internet-based CBT has been developed to improve accessibility to patients who are unable to engage with traditional CBT.[36] Patients with RA have shown improvements in quality of life and self-efficacy after pain-focused Internet-based CBT, but evidence has not shown improvements in disability, mood, or pain.[37–39]

Spondyloarthritides

There are little data looking at CBT in SpA specifically. One small study of patients with ankylosing spondylitis (AS) treated with CBT showed a moderate beneficial effect on subjective ratings of pain.[40] Fibromyalgia shows significant overlap with psoriatic arthritis (PsA) and other forms of SpA, and has been shown to see short- and long-term improvement in pain with pain-directed CBT.[27,41–43] CBT has shown benefit in chronic pain generally but proving its efficacy in SpA requires further study.[44,45]

MINDFULNESS-BASED INTERVENTIONS

MBIs typically take the form of training programs that seek to equip patients with the tools to practice nonjudgmental awareness of one's present experience and encourage openness, curiosity, and acceptance of that experience.[46] The underlying principal is to reduce reactivity to unpleasant internal phenomenon and promote a reflective engagement with one's experience.[46] Two of the most common MBIs are mindfulness-based stress reduction (MBSR) and mindfulness-based cognitive therapy (MBCT), which typically follow an 8-week format of weekly meetings that incorporate meditation and talk-therapy to build skills that can continue to be practiced at home.[46]

Rheumatoid Arthritis

Several forms of MBI have demonstrated improvement on pain in patients with RA. Internal family systems therapy and mindful awareness and acceptance therapy have directly measured improvement in pain scores in this population.[24,47,48] These interventions take different approaches to a similar goal, internal family systems focusing on fostering an internal dialogue by treating one's parts as subpersonalities, and mindful awareness and acceptance therapy focusing on building skills to reduce the effect of pain and enhance positive affect.[47,49] A head-to-head trial of mindful awareness and acceptance therapy against CBT in patients with RA found that CBT offered a greater effect on pain except for in patients with comorbid depression, which showed greater effect from mindful awareness and acceptance therapy.[48]

Studies of MBSR in patients with RA have shown improvements in self-efficacy, well-being as measured by the Psychological Well-Being Scales, patient global assessment score, tender joint count, swollen joint count, and disease activity.[14,50,51] Although these studies did not measure effect on pain directly, pain is an important contributor to patient global assessment, providing a potential proxy for pain's measure.[52]

There is a paucity of evidence regarding the effect of MBCT on pain directly in patients with RA. In fact, many MBCT trials on patients with chronic pain focus on measuring changes in patients' interactions with pain (eg, pain catastrophizing, pain acceptance) rather than direct pain scale.[53,54] MBCT does show improved patient interaction with pain and several measures of self-efficacy (eg, control over disease) in cases of chronic pain.[53–55] An Internet-delivered module of MBCT has demonstrated similar benefit, expanding access and reducing barriers to engagement.[55] Dalili and Bayazi[56] showed improvement in patients with RA after MBCT with regard to illness perception as measured by the Illness Perception Questionnaire and psychological symptoms in patients with RA but did not measure pain outcomes directly.

Spondyloarthritis

Data on MBIs, specifically on patients with SpA, are limited, and neither MBSR nor MBCT have been evaluated in a randomized trial setting in patients with SpA. A study of mixed inflammatory arthritis patients including patients with AS and PsA treated with an MBI called Vitality Training Programme (a program that incorporated 15 weeks of semiweekly therapy and a 6-month "booster" session to incorporate creativity into mindfulness-based teaching) showed evidence of significantly improved self-efficacy, but not pain.[57]

Illness perception, which is improved by MBCT in patients with RA, is correlated with back pain in patients with axial spondyloarthropathy (AxSpA).[56,58] If the gains in illness perception are generalizable to the SpA population, MBCT may prove an effective avenue of pain control in SpA. A case-report describes one patient with PsA who experienced subjectively improved pain control and ability to manage pain 6 months after an 8-week MBSR course.[59] Although this report did not conduct an objective comparison of pretreatment and post-treatment measures, in the absence of additional evidence of MBIs effect in SpA, it provides guidance toward potentially fruitful avenues of further investigation.

PATIENT EDUCATION

Disease-focused PE provides tools for patients to develop self-management skills, use lifestyle changes, and claim responsibility for day-to-day symptom management.[60] EULAR recommends disease-centered education routinely in inflammatory arthritis.[61]

Rheumatoid Arthritis

Data are conflicting on whether patients with RA derive significant improvement in pain and self-efficacy from disease-based PE.[12,62–64] When improvements in pain are observed after disease-based PE the effect size is generally smaller than that of CBT or MBI.[12,65] Structured self-management programs that incorporate self-regulation and coping tools teaching with PE show greater improvements in pain compared with group education alone.[14]

Programs such as the Arthritis Self-Management Program and Self-Management Arthritis Relief Therapy mail-based program promote increased self-efficacy by providing tools for patients to engage with their disease through teaching a combination of behavioral and discussion-based techniques.[14,15,66,67] Their use has been shown to significantly improve pain, disability, and self-efficacy in patients with RA.[67,68] The benefit of these programs is long standing, with one study suggesting that the Arthritis Self-Management Program may show pain benefit for 4 years after completion.[69] The generalizability of this finding is questionable because a systematic review of 31 randomized controlled trials evaluating PE in RA found no significant effect on pain at follow-up.[30] Whether that loss of long-term effect is caused by heterogeneity of PE programs or reversion to a mean is difficult to determine based on the available evidence.

Spondyloarthritis

There is a dearth of evidence regarding the effect of PE on pain in SpA.[61,70] What evidence does exist suggests that there is a significant unmet need for SpA-based PE as measured by an Educational Needs Assessment Tool.[70,71] Generally, women with inflammatory arthritis display an increased desire for education over men.[70,72] Mixed cohorts of patients with assorted inflammatory arthritides found small short-term improvements in pain and self-efficacy after PE programs.[73,74] Further study into effective forms of PE in SpA may aid with program selection to achieve optimal effect.

BIOFEEDBACK

Biofeedback is a form of therapy in which patients are provided with information regarding the intensity of a physiologic response under autonomic control to develop the ability to modulate that response.[12,34] Biofeedback, with and without CBT, has been shown to increase self-efficacy in nonspecific chronic pain.[75]

Rheumatoid Arthritis

Thermal biofeedback provides skin temperature information to patients to assist with development of control over peripheral temperature via vasodilation.[76] Effectively developing this ability requires training, but when focused on temperature elevation at their most painful joint, patients with RA have shown improved measures of pain.[32,34,76,77] Technological advancement continues to introduce new modalities through which to deliver biofeedback with one study of virtual reality–based biofeedback in a small, RA-predominant cohort of patients with rheumatologic disease showing improved pain scores after virtual reality biofeedback training.[78]

Spondyloarthritis

As with many other nonpharmacologic interventions, there is a paucity of SpA-specific research regarding biofeedback. Conflicting evidence exists regarding the efficacy of biofeedback in controlling psoriatic skin disease, but some studies have shown that biofeedback, either with or without concomitant CBT, have improved skin disease in psoriasis subjectively and as measured by Psoriasis Area and Severity Index.[79–81] Skin and joint disease activity do not correlate well in psoriatic disease, but skin activity is included in some experimental measures of disease activity in PsA, and biofeedback's potential efficacy in skin disease provides an open avenue for further investigation in its effect on rheumatic manifestations of psoriatic disease.[82]

EXERCISE AND PHYSICAL ACTIVITY

Physical activity and exercise are routinely recommended in the treatment of RA, PsA, and AxSpA.[2,9,83] The benefits of exercise extend beyond pain associated with inflammatory arthritis, but the appreciable benefit it can offer to patients with inflammatory arthritis pain can serve as an additional motivation to engage with this generally health-enhancing behavior. In patients with chronic pain exercise should follow a slow and gradual progression to reduce the risk for flares of pain that may lead to loss of program engagement.[30]

Rheumatoid Arthritis

Aerobic exercise has shown a small but significant improvement in pain in patients with RA, whereas resistance training showed a statistically insignificant trend in the same direction.[84–86] Under supervised conditions these programs were not found to cause deleterious effects, such as short-term increased pain, debility, or joint damage.[84] A combination of modalities has been shown to offer long-lasting benefit, with one mixed aerobic exercise and resistance training program combined with weekly group-based discussions showing an improvement in pain that persisted at 2-year follow-up.[87] Low-impact modalities, such as hydrotherapy, yoga, and tai chi, have conflicting evidence that shows either no or small effects on pain scores in patients with RA.[12,88]

Spondyloarthritis

Although some physical activity is beneficial in SpA, patients with AS with jobs requiring dynamic flexibility consisting of bending, twisting, stretching, and reaching showed greater functional limitations compared with patients without those demands.[89] Exercise programs have low-quality evidence for pain control in SpA, although they can show improvement in physical function and disease activity.[89,90] The benefits offered by exercise are generally greater when performed in a supervised group setting, such as physiotherapy, as opposed to independent at home.[89] Intensive, residential spa-based multidisciplinary exercise therapy showed strong results that persisted for 6 months, although the time and cost required for these therapies may prove prohibitive for some patients.[90] Low-impact exercise modalities, such as hydrotherapy and Baduanjin (a form of mindfulness-based physical movement akin to tai chi) have shown improvement in patient-reported pain in patients with AS, although the amount of evidence is limited.[91,92]

MASSAGE

Massage is a form of manual physical manipulation that seeks to improve pain and physical function through reducing muscle tension, increasing circulation, and stimulating the parasympathetic system.[12] It has been shown to improve pain scores immediately after intervention in noninflammatory chronic pain conditions, although there is little support for long-term effect.[93]

Rheumatoid Arthritis

Joint-targeted aromatherapy massage showed improvement in pain scores after 6 weeks of treatment in patients with RA, although there was no long-term follow-up.[94] Similar effects on pain have been seen in adult and juvenile RA after shorter courses of massage therapy, sometimes to near resolution immediately postintervention, although again, these studies lack long-term follow-up data.[94–96] Although patients with RA have derived pain benefits in hand- and knee-targeted massage, foot-targeted massage has not demonstrated similar effect.[94,95,97] The intensity of massage may be related to the effect size, because moderate-intensity massage has been shown to be superior to light massage in improving pain.[95] There is ancillary benefit to range of motion, mood, and anxiety after massage.[93] The long-term effect of massage on these domains has not been well-studied in this population and warrants further investigation.

Spondyloarthritis

Case and small cohort studies have shown improvements in pain, fatigue, and stiffness in patients with AS.[98,99] Deep tissue massage showed a comparatively large improvement in lower back pain in patients with AS as compared with lower intensity therapeutic massage.[99] Massage has not been studied specifically in patients with other SpAs, but is recommended conditionally by the American College of Rheumatology based on data supporting its use in osteoarthritis and RA.[83,100] There have been case reports that describes disastrous cervical spinal cord injury in patients with AS during massage leading to paralysis and death, but these are rare events and massage is generally considered safe when medical conditions are disclosed and appropriate precautions are taken (eg, avoiding the cervical area in patients with AS or atlantoaxial instability).[101–103]

ORTHOTICS/SPLINTS

On the whole, evidence for the efficacy of supportive garments, such as wrist splints or foot orthoses, in inflammatory arthritis is conflicting.[104,105]

Rheumatoid Arthritis

Studies have showed that resting and active wrist splinting offers little benefit in the short to medium term in patients with RA.[104] Despite this lack of improvement, patients generally prefer to continue wearing wrist splints after 2 months of use.[104] A single, small study with longer follow-up has shown significant improvement in hand pain that emerged at 90 days of treatment with night splinting in patients with RA, raising the possibility that the effect is simply delayed rather than not present.[106] In patients with RA, certain types of orthotics (extradepth shoes with semirigid insoles) have shown improved pain when walking and climbing stairs, and more pain-free walking time compared with control subjects, whereas other types of orthotics have shown no improvement.[104,105]

Spondyloarthritis

There is no evidence evaluating the use of orthoses in patients with SpA.[107,108] Splinting has been used in juvenile PsA with positive effect on maintaining joint position, but its effect on pain was not directly evaluated.[109]

BALNEOTHERAPY

Balneotherapy (also known as spa therapy or mineral baths) involves soaking in an indoor pool at a temperature between 31°C and 36°C and is sometimes combined with heated mud or other natural peloid packs.[110,111] Balneotherapy is generally safe and has been used for centuries as part of treatment of orthopedic and musculoskeletal conditions.[110]

Rheumatoid Arthritis

There is inconsistent evidence regarding pain improvement after balneotherapy in patients with RA.[112] Effect seems influenced by selection of liquid medium, with mineral baths showing significant improvement in pain that persisted at 8 weeks, and radon-carbon dioxin baths showing delayed improvement in pain that only surfaced 6 months after therapy, whereas Dead Sea salt water and tap water baths did not show a similar effect.[110] The quality of evidence supporting these findings is low, hampered by small sample sizes and methodologic flaws (eg, lack of intention to treat analysis, lack of double blinding).[110]

Spondyloarthritis

Balneotherapy has been found to improve pain and mobility in patients with AxSpA to a greater and more consistent degree when compared with patients with peripheral inflammatory arthritis.[111] Patients with AS and PsA have shown balneotherapy to be an effective adjuvant for pain treatment, whereas patients with enteropathic arthritis have shown improvements in global activity scores.[111,113] Selection of balneotherapy modality is less well associated with degree of effect in SpA as compared with RA.[111] The benefits of balneotherapy in SpA disappear over 6 to 15 months.[89] It should be noted that balneotherapy should be avoided in acute arthritides, such as reactive or gouty arthritis.[111]

ACUPUNCTURE

Acupuncture is a millennia-old practice that originated in ancient China.[114] It operates on the principle that energy called *qi* flows through the body and can cause illness through imbalance.[114] The goal of acupuncture is to correct the flow of *qi* along channels called meridians with the use of hair thin needles placed in the skin.[114] In chronic pain generally there is conflicting evidence for the efficacy of acupuncture.[115,116] Although acupuncture is generally safe, there are reports of rare, potentially serious complications of acupuncture, such as infection or, in a worst-case scenario, death secondary to pneumothorax, making trained, experienced practitioner selection particularly important.[114]

Rheumatoid Arthritis

The study of acupuncture in patients with RA is more robust in the Chinese population than in the Western world.[117] Western-focused systematic reviews have found conflicting evidence regarding acupuncture's effectiveness in controlling pain in patients with RA.[118,119] The quality and number of western studies available for review was limited.[118,119] A similar systematic review incorporating Chinese studies showed a preponderance of reported improvements in pain in Chinese, but not western studies, which may indicate a lack of generalizability.[117]

More recently, a well-powered randomized controlled trial of verum (traditional, meridian based) acupuncture against sham (nonmeridian based) acupuncture and a waiting list nontreatment group showed improvement in pain in sham and verum acupuncture, with a dramatically increased degree of effect in verum-arm patients.[120] Verum acupuncture via nontraditional means, such as laser or bee venom therapy, has demonstrated improvements in pain, suggesting the location of therapy is an important part of the observed effect.[121,122] The long-term effect of acupuncture after completion is unclear, as is the duration of treatment necessary to consistently see effect, although benefit has been observed after 4 weeks of twice-weekly treatment, and 4 to 10 sessions should be considered an adequate trial.[117,120,123]

Spondyloarthritis

The American College of Rheumatology conditionally recommends acupuncture in patients with PsA because of low-quality case-report-level evidence of its benefit.[83,124] Systematic reviews have found that patients with fibromyalgia find improvements in pain after acupuncture, an effect that may be generalizable to some degree in patients with PsA based on the high prevalence of fibromyalgia in that population.[42,125] Again, studies in western literature are lacking with regard to acupuncture in patients with other types of SpA.

SLEEP

Poor sleep and chronic pain have a bidirectional relationship, in which the exacerbation of one condition often contributes to exacerbation of the other.[126] Addressing sleep, even in the absence of chronic pain, involves evaluation of physiologic disorders and engagement with cognitive and behavioral therapies that require proactive home practice.[126]

Rheumatoid Arthritis

There is a high prevalence of sleep disturbance (45%–70%) in patients with RA, with patients experiencing higher disease activity demonstrating poorer quality sleep.[127–129] Poorer quality sleep reduces pain threshold and increases pain intensity in patients with RA.[127,130] Sleep is, in turn, negatively affected by RA-associated pain, with up to 42% of that sleep disturbance attributable to RA when compared with noninflammatory disease matched control subjects.[131]

Pharmacotherapy for sleep disturbance lacks consensus or evidence-based algorithms, but nonpharmacologic sleep treatments have been shown to offer large improvements in sleep quality in patients with chronic pain.[127,132] Exercise and biofeedback-based relaxation techniques have shown improvements in sleep quality in patients with RA, and insomnia-focused CBT in patients with RA is currently being investigated, supported by evidence that shows effectiveness in patients with chronic pain.[77,132–134] Brief Behavioral Treatment for Insomnia is another psychological therapy that involves fewer, shorter sessions than CBT and has shown sleep improvement in cases of insomnia, but has not been studied in inflammatory arthritis specifically.[12,135]

Spondyloarthritis

Patients with SpA experience significantly more frequent sleep disturbance than control populations, with poor quality sleep in 84% of patients with PsA and 80% of patients with AS.[136–138] Pain and degree of sleep disturbance are directly linked in PsA, although causality is difficult to determine.[139,140] Nighttime pain in inflammatory arthritis creates a feedback loop with sleep disturbance, and patients with AxSpA experience more subjectively severe nighttime stiffness and pain as compared with patients with RA.[141]

Treatments to improve sleep quality in SpA have not been well assessed. Exercise has been shown to improve sleep quality in patients with AxSpA, although the evidence for long-term effect is mixed, and the size of the effect seems to be small.[136,142]

DEPRESSION

Depression is a common comorbidity in patients with RA and SpA, with prevalence far outstripping that of a healthy age-matched population.[143–145] Depression negatively influences pain experience and interferes with coping.[12] Complementarily, pain is one of the strongest predictors of depression in RA, and patients with inflammatory arthritis with comorbid anxiety and depression are more likely to experience increased symptom burden including pain.[12] Depression treatment is beyond the scope of this review but referral for treatment of comorbid depression synergistically improves pain management in patients with inflammatory arthritis.

INEFFECTIVE THERAPIES
Magnets

Static magnet therapy is marketed as providing pain relief in chronic pain conditions, and one survey of patients with RA, osteoarthritis, and fibromyalgia suggests that up to 28% of that pooled cohort has trialed static magnetic therapy.[146] Systematic review of comparable, randomized, placebo-controlled studies of static magnets in chronic pain did not provide evidence of analgesic benefit.[147] Studies evaluating static magnet therapy in patients with RA specifically showed a difference in baseline versus 4-week pain scores in patients with unipolar and quadrapolar static magnetic field therapy for the knee without any statistical significance between the two.[148] These interventions were not compared with sham treatment, limiting the evaluation of potential placebo effect.[148] Static magnet therapy has not been directly evaluated in SpA, but in the absence of evidence for its efficacy in other chronic pain conditions there is little rationale for its use unless the evidence base changes.

Chiropractic

There is inadequate evidence to support the effectiveness of chiropractic adjustment in controlling pain in inflammatory arthritis, although patient satisfaction is reportedly higher in chiropractic intervention than acupuncture, osteopathic medicine, and massage.[30] Given the lack of evidence for improved outcomes in chiropractic treatment, the consequences of poorly controlled SpA or RA can lead to disastrous results during chiropractic adjustment, such as vertebral fracture or dislocation.[102,149,150] Patients with inflammatory arthritis should undergo chiropractic adjustment, particularly involving the cervical spine, with exceptional caution.

SUMMARY

Nonpharmacologic modalities offer a diverse bevy of options to address pain in inflammatory arthritis, allowing patients and providers to engage in shared decision making to find options that are enticing and accessible. Many nonpharmacologic interventions offer the added benefit of developing self-efficacy by offering opportunities for patients to claim ownership over management of the symptoms of their disease. Self-efficacy potentiates the effect of self-directed nonpharmacologic interventions, creating a virtuous cycle of building effective patient self-management.

There is a general paucity of research regarding nonpharmacologic treatment effects on pain in SpA, a ripe opportunity to discover differential effects between SpA and RA as seen with balneotherapy. Effective nonpharmacologic interventions effect on patients' pain, and the effect's duration (when studied) was typically less than 12 months. Some interventions that have used booster sessions have shown extension of that effect, suggesting that nonpharmacologic interventions require maintenance in chronic diseases, much like their pharmacologic counterparts.

CLINICS CARE POINTS

- It is of paramount importance to have an action plan that includes multidisciplinary, integrative management of pain in patients with inflammatory arthritis.
- There is evidence for improved pain in patients with RA with CBT, MBI, biofeedback, aerobic or combined exercise, massage, hand splints, orthotics, and balneotherapy.
- There is evidence for improved pain in patients with SpA with physiotherapy, massage, and balneotherapy.
- Investigation has been unable to demonstrate strong evidence of impact on pain with static magnet therapy or chiropractic adjustment in patients with SpA or RA.
- Addressing chronic pain modulating issues, such as sleep and depression, is an important part of pain management in patients with inflammatory arthritis.

DISCLOSURE

No disclosure.

REFERENCES

1. Bergman MJ. Social and economic impact of inflammatory arthritis. Postgrad Med 2006;(Spec No):5–11.
2. Borenstein D, Altman R, Bello A, et al. Report of the American College of Rheumatology Pain Management Task Force. Arthritis Care Res 2010;62(5):590–9.
3. Heiberg T, Finset A, Uhlig T, et al. Seven year changes in health status and priorities for improvement of health in patients with rheumatoid arthritis. Ann Rheum Dis 2005;64(2):191–5.
4. Ten Klooster PM, Veehof MM, Taal E, et al. Changes in priorities for improvement in patients with rheumatoid arthritis during 1 year of anti-tumour necrosis factor treatment. Ann Rheum Dis 2007;66(11):1485–90.
5. Lee YC. Effect and treatment of chronic pain in inflammatory arthritis. Curr Rheumatol Rep 2013;15(1). https://doi.org/10.1007/s11926-012-0300-4.
6. Hamilton-West KE, Quine L. Living with ankylosing spondylitis: the patient's perspective. J Health Psychol 2009;14(6):820–30.
7. Husni ME, Merola JF, Davin S. The psychosocial burden of psoriatic arthritis. Semin Arthritis Rheum 2017;47(3):351–60.
8. Singh JA, Saag KG, Bridges SL, et al. 2015 American College of Rheumatology Guideline for the Treatment of Rheumatoid Arthritis. Arthritis Care Res (Hoboken) 2016;68(1):1–25.
9. Ward MM, Deodhar A, Gensler LS, et al. 2019 Update of the American College of Rheumatology/Spondylitis Association of America/Spondyloarthritis Research and Treatment Network Recommendations for the Treatment of Ankylosing Spondylitis and Nonradiographic Axial Spondyloarthritis. Arthritis Rheumatol 2019;71(10):1599–613.
10. Kidd BL, Langford RM, Wodehouse T. Current approaches in the treatment of arthritic pain. Arthritis Res Ther 2007;9(3):1–7.
11. van de Laar M. Pain treatment in arthritis-related pain: beyond NSAIDs. Open Rheumatol J 2012;6(1):320–30.
12. Nicassio PM. Psychosocial factors in arthritis: perspectives on adjustment and management. Switzerland: Springer International Publishing; 2015. Available at: https://books.google.com/books?id=QNYLCwAAQBAJ.
13. Bandura A. Self-efficacy: toward a unifying theory of behavioral change. Psychol Rev 1977;84(2):191–215.
14. DiRenzo D, Finan P. Self-efficacy and the role of non-pharmacologic treatment strategies to improve pain and affect in arthritis. Curr Treat Options Rheumatol 2019;5(2):168–78.
15. Marks R, Allegrante JP, Lorig K. A review and synthesis of research evidence for self-efficacy-enhancing interventions for reducing chronic disability: implications for health education practice (part II). Health Promot Pract 2005;6(2):148–56.
16. O'Leary A, Shoor S, Lorig K, et al. A cognitive-behavioral treatment for rheumatoid arthritis. Health Psychol 1988;7(6):527–44.
17. O'Leary A. Self-efficacy and health. Behav Res Ther 1985;23(4):437–51.
18. Meredith P, Strong J, Feeney JA. Adult attachment, anxiety, and pain self-efficacy as predictors of pain intensity and disability. Pain 2006;123(1–2):146–54.

19. Knittle KP, De Gucht V, Hurkmans EJ, et al. Effect of self-efficacy and physical activity goal achievement on arthritis pain and quality of life in patients with rheumatoid arthritis. Arthritis Care Res 2011;63(11):1613–9.

20. Liu L, Xu N, Wang L. Moderating role of self-efficacy on the associations of social support with depressive and anxiety symptoms in Chinese patients with rheumatoid arthritis. Neuropsychiatr Dis Treat 2017;13:2141–50.

21. Somers TJ, Wren AA, Shelby RA. The context of pain in arthritis: self-efficacy for managing pain and other symptoms. Curr Pain Headache Rep 2012;16(6):502–8.

22. Martinez-Calderon J, Meeus M, Struyf F, et al. The role of self-efficacy in pain intensity, function, psychological factors, health behaviors, and quality of life in people with rheumatoid arthritis: a systematic review. Physiother Theory Pract 2020;36(1):21–37.

23. Lenker SL, Lorig K, Gallagher D. Reasons for the lack of association between changes in health behavior and improved health status: an exploratory study. Patient Educ Couns 1984;6(2):69–72.

24. DiRenzo D, Crespo-Bosque M, Gould N, et al. Systematic review and meta-analysis: mindfulness-based interventions for rheumatoid arthritis. Curr Rheumatol Rep 2018;20(12):1–19.

25. Finney Rutten LJ, Hesse BW, St. Sauver JL, et al. Health self-efficacy among populations with multiple chronic conditions: the value of patient-centered communication. Adv Ther 2016;33(8):1440–51.

26. Marks R. Self-efficacy and arthritis disability: an updated synthesis of the evidence base and its relevance to optimal patient care. Health Psychol Open 2014;1. https://doi.org/10.1177/2055102914564582.

27. Callahan LF, Shreffler JH, Altpeter M, et al. Evaluation of group and self-directed formats of the arthritis foundation's Walk With Ease program. Arthritis Care Res 2011;63(8):1098–107.

28. Sharpe L. Psychosocial management of chronic pain in patients with rheumatoid arthritis: challenges and solutions. J Pain Res 2016;9:137–46.

29. Nash VR, Ponto J, Townsend C, et al. Cognitive behavioral therapy, self-efficacy, and depression in persons with chronic pain. Pain Manag Nurs 2013;14(4):e236–43.

30. Cunningham NR, Kashikar-Zuck S. Nonpharmacological treatment of pain in rheumatic diseases and other musculoskeletal pain conditions. Curr Rheumatol Rep 2013;15(2):1–14.

31. Knittle K, Maes S, De Gucht V. Psychological interventions for rheumatoid arthritis: examining the role of self-regulation with a systematic review and meta-analysis of randomized controlled trials. Arthritis Care Res 2010;62(10):1460–72.

32. Astin JA, Beckner W, Soeken K, et al. Psychological interventions for rheumatoid arthritis: a meta-analysis of randomized controlled trials. Arthritis Care Res 2002;47(3):291–302.

33. Prothero L, Barley E, Galloway J, et al. The evidence base for psychological interventions for rheumatoid arthritis: a systematic review of reviews. Int J Nurs Stud 2018;82(August 2017):20–9.

34. Dissanayake RK, Bertouch JV. Psychosocial interventions as adjunct therapy for patients with rheumatoid arthritis: a systematic review. Int J Rheum Dis 2010;13(4):324–34.

35. Evers AWM, Kraaimaat FW, Van Riel PLCM, et al. Tailored cognitive-behavioral therapy in early rheumatoid arthritis for patients at risk: a randomized controlled trial. Pain 2002;100(1–2):141–53.
36. Rini C, Porter LS, Somers TJ, et al. Retaining critical therapeutic elements of behavioral interventions translated for delivery via the Internet: recommendations and an example using pain coping skills training. J Med Internet Res 2014;16(12):1–14.
37. Ferwerda M, Van Beugen S, Van Middendorp H, et al. A tailored-guided internet-based cognitive-behavioral intervention for patients with rheumatoid arthritis as an adjunct to standard rheumatological care: results of a randomized controlled trial. Pain 2017;158(5):868–78.
38. Shigaki CL, Smarr KL, Siva C, et al. RAHelp: an online intervention for individuals with rheumatoid arthritis. Arthritis Care Res 2013;65(10):1573–81.
39. Trudeau KJ, Pujol LA, DasMahapatra P, et al. A randomized controlled trial of an online self-management program for adults with arthritis pain. J Behav Med 2015;38(3):483–96.
40. Basler HD, Rehfisch HP. Cognitive-behavioral therapy in patients with ankylosing spondylitis in a German self-help organization. J Psychosom Res 1991;35(2–3):345–54.
41. Bernardy K, Füber N, Köllner V, et al. Efficacy of cognitive-behavioral therapies in fibromyalgia syndrome: a systematic review and metaanalysis of randomized controlled trials. J Rheumatol 2010;37(10):1991–2005.
42. Magrey MN, Antonelli M, James N, et al. High frequency of fibromyalgia in patients with psoriatic arthritis: a pilot study. Arthritis 2013;2013:1–4.
43. Wach J, Letroublon MC, Coury F, et al. Fibromyalgia in spondyloarthritis: effect on disease activity assessment in clinical practice. J Rheumatol 2016;43(11):2056–63.
44. Morley S, Eccleston C, Williams A. Systematic review and meta-analysis of randomized controlled trials of cognitive behaviour therapy and behaviour therapy for chronic pain in adults, excluding headache. Pain 1999;80(1–2):1–13.
45. Batko B. Patient-centered care in psoriatic arthritis: a perspective on inflammation, disease activity, and psychosocial factors. J Clin Med 2020;9(10):3103.
46. Hofmann SG, Gómez AF. Mindfulness-based interventions for anxiety and depression. Psychiatr Clin North Am 2017;40(4):739–49.
47. Shadick NA, Sowell NF, Frits ML, et al. A randomized controlled trial of an internal family systems-based psychotherapeutic intervention on outcomes in rheumatoid arthritis: a proof-of-concept study. J Rheumatol 2013;40(11):1831–41.
48. Zautra AJ, Davis MC, Reich JW, et al. Comparison of cognitive behavioral and mindfulness meditation interventions on adaptation to rheumatoid arthritis for patients with and without history of recurrent depression. J Consult Clin Psychol 2008;76(3):408–21.
49. Davis MC, Zautra AJ, Wolf LD, et al. Mindfulness and cognitive-behavioral interventions for chronic pain: differential effects on daily pain reactivity and stress reactivity. J Consult Clin Psychol 2015;83(1):24–35.
50. Fogarty FA, Booth RJ, Gamble GD, et al. The effect of mindfulness-based stress reduction on disease activity in people with rheumatoid arthritis: a randomised controlled trial. Ann Rheum Dis 2015;74(2):472–4.
51. Pradhan EK, Baumgarten M, Langenberg P, et al. Effect of mindfulness-based stress reduction in rheumatoid arthritis patients. Arthritis Care Res 2007;57(7):1134–42.

52. Challa DNV, Crowson CS, Davis JM. The Patient Global Assessment of Disease Activity in rheumatoid arthritis: identification of underlying latent factors. Rheumatol Ther 2017;4(1):201–8.

53. de Jong M, Lazar SW, Hug K, et al. Effects of mindfulness-based cognitive therapy on body awareness in patients with chronic pain and comorbid depression. Front Psychol 2016;7. https://doi.org/10.3389/fpsyg.2016.00967.

54. Moore KM, Martin ME. Using MBCT in a chronic pain setting: a qualitative analysis of participants' experiences. Mindfulness (N Y) 2015;6(5):1129–36.

55. Dowd H, Hogan MJ, McGuire BE, et al. Comparison of an online mindfulness-based cognitive therapy intervention with online pain management psychoeducation: a randomized controlled study. Clin J Pain 2015;31(6):517–27.

56. Dalili Z, Bayazi MH. The effectiveness of mindfulness-based cognitive therapy on the illness perception and psychological symptoms in patients with rheumatoid arthritis. Complement Ther Clin Pract 2019;34:139–44.

57. Zangi HA, Mowinckel P, Finset A, et al. A mindfulness-based group intervention to reduce psychological distress and fatigue in patients with inflammatory rheumatic joint diseases: a randomised controlled trial. Ann Rheum Dis 2012;71(6):911–7.

58. van Lunteren M, Scharloo M, Ez-Zaitouni Z, et al. The impact of illness perceptions and coping on the association between back pain and health outcomes in patients suspected of having axial spondyloarthritis: data from the SPondyloArthritis Caught Early Cohort. Arthritis Care Res 2018;70(12):1829–39.

59. Hawtin H, Sullivan C. Experiences of mindfulness training in living with rheumatic disease: an interpretative phenomenological analysis. Br J Occup Ther 2011;74(3):137.

60. Barlow J, Wright C, Sheasby J, et al. Self-management approaches for people with chronic conditions: a review. Patient Educ Couns 2002;48(2):177–87.

61. Zangi HA, Ndosi M, Adams J, et al. EULAR recommendations for patient education for people with inflammatory arthritis. Ann Rheum Dis 2015;74(6):954–62.

62. Barsky AJ, Ahern DK, Orav EJ, et al. A randomized trial of three psychosocial treatments for the symptoms of rheumatoid arthritis. Semin Arthritis Rheum 2010;40(3):222–32.

63. Riemsma RP, Taal E, Kirwan JR, et al. Systematic review of rheumatoid arthritis patient education. Arthritis Care Res 2004;51(6):1045–59.

64. Ndosi M, Johnson D, Young T, et al. Effects of needs-based patient education on self-efficacy and health outcomes in people with rheumatoid arthritis: a multicentre, single blind, randomised controlled trial. Ann Rheum Dis 2016;75(6):1126–32.

65. Hammond A, Bryan J, Hardy A. Effects of a modular behavioural arthritis education programme: a pragmatic parallel-group randomized controlled trial. Rheumatology 2008;47(11):1712–8.

66. Lorig KR, Ritter PL, Laurent DD, et al. Long-term randomized controlled trials of tailored-print and small-group arthritis self-management interventions. Med Care 2004;42(4):346–54.

67. Conn DL, Pan Y, Easley KA, et al. The effect of the Arthritis Self-Management Program on outcome in African Americans with rheumatoid arthritis served by a public hospital. Clin Rheumatol 2013;32(1):49–59.

68. Lorig KR, Sobel DS, Ritter PL, et al. Effect of a self-management program on patients with chronic disease. Eff Clin Pract 2001;4(6):256–62.

69. Lorig KR, Mazonson PD, Holman HR. Evidence suggesting that health education for self-management in patients with chronic arthritis has sustained health benefits while reducing health care costs. Arthritis Rheum 1993;36(4):439–46.
70. Haglund E, Bremander A, Bergman S, et al. Educational needs in patients with spondyloarthritis in Sweden: a mixed-methods study. BMC Musculoskelet Disord 2017;18(1):1–9.
71. Lubrano E, Helliwell P, Moreno P, et al. The assessment of knowledge in ankylosing spondylitis patients by a self-administered questionnaire. Br J Rheumatol 1998;37(4):437–41.
72. Drăgoi R, Ndosi M, Sadlonova M, et al. Patient education, disease activity and physical. Arthritis Res Ther 2013. https://doi.org/10.1186/ar4339.
73. Rudd RE, Blanch DC, Gall V, et al. A randomized controlled trial of an intervention to reduce low literacy barriers in inflammatory arthritis management. Patient Educ Couns 2009;75(3):334–9.
74. Grønning K, Rannestad T, Skomsvoll JF, et al. Long-term effects of a nurse-led group and individual patient education programme for patients with chronic inflammatory polyarthritis: a randomised controlled trial. J Clin Nurs 2014;23(7–8):1005–17.
75. Gatchel RJ, Robinson RC, Pulliam C, et al. Biofeedback with pain patients: evidence for its effectiveness. Semin Pain Med 2003;1(2):55–66.
76. Bradley LA, Young LD, Anderson KO, et al. Effects of psychological therapy on pain behavior of rheumatoid arthritis patients. Treatment outcome and six-month followup. Arthritis Rheum 1987;30(10):1105–14.
77. Achterberg J, McGraw P, Lawlis GF. Rheumatoid arthritis: a study of relaxation and temperature biofeedback training as an adjunctive therapy. Biofeedback Self Regul 1981;6(2):207–23.
78. Venuturupalli RS, Chu T, Vicari M, et al. Virtual reality–based biofeedback and guided meditation in rheumatology: a pilot study. ACR Open Rheumatol 2019;1(10):667–75.
79. Qureshi AA, Awosika O, Baruffi F, et al. Psychological therapies in management of psoriatic skin disease: a systematic review. Am J Clin Dermatol 2019;20(5):607–24.
80. Keinan G, Segal A, Gal U, et al. Stress management for psoriasis patients: the effectiveness of biofeedback and relaxation techniques. Stress Med 1995;11(1):235–41.
81. Piaserico S, Marinello E, Dessi A, et al. Efficacy of biofeedback and cognitive-behavioural therapy in psoriatic patients: a single-blind, randomized and controlled study with added narrow-band ultraviolet B therapy. Acta Derm Venereol 2016;96(5):91–5.
82. Wong PCH, Leung YY, Li EK, et al. Measuring disease activity in psoriatic arthritis. Int J Rheumatol 2012;2012. https://doi.org/10.1155/2012/839425.
83. Singh JA, Guyatt G, Ogdie A, et al. Special article: 2018 American College of Rheumatology/National Psoriasis Foundation guideline for the treatment of psoriatic arthritis. Arthritis Rheumatol 2019;71(1):5–32.
84. Hurkmans EJ, Maes S, de Gucht V, et al. Motivation as a determinant of physical activity in patients with rheumatoid arthritis. Arthritis Care Res (Hoboken) 2010;62(3):371–7.
85. Ekelman BA, Hooker L, Davis A, et al. Occupational therapy interventions for adults with rheumatoid arthritis: an appraisal of the evidence. Occup Ther Heal Care 2014;28(4):347–61.

86. Baillet A, Vaillant M, Guinot M, et al. Efficacy of resistance exercises in rheumatoid arthritis: meta-analysis of randomized controlled trials. Rheumatology 2012; 51(3):519–27.

87. Löfgren M, Opava CH, Demmelmaier I, et al. Long-term, health-enhancing physical activity is associated with reduction of pain but not pain sensitivity or improved exercise-induced hypoalgesia in persons with rheumatoid arthritis. Arthritis Res Ther 2018;20(1):1–9.

88. Al-Qubaeissy KY, Fatoye FA, Goodwin PC, et al. The effectiveness of hydrotherapy in the management of rheumatoid arthritis: a systematic review. Musculoskeletal Care 2013;11(1):3–18.

89. Reimold AM, Chandran V. Nonpharmacologic therapies in spondyloarthritis. Best Pract Res Clin Rheumatol 2014;28(5):779–92.

90. O'Dwyer T, O'Shea F, Wilson F. Exercise therapy for spondyloarthritis: a systematic review. Rheumatol Int 2014;34(7):887–902.

91. Martin M, Gilbert A, Jeffries C. OP0279-HPR A national survey of the utilisation and experience of hydrotherapy in the management of axial spondyloarthritis: the patients' perspective. Ann Rheum Dis 2018;77(Suppl 2):187–8.

92. Zou L, Yeung A, Quan X, et al. A systematic review and meta-analysis of mindfulness-based (Baduanjin) exercise for alleviating musculoskeletal pain and improving sleep quality in people with chronic diseases. Int J Environ Res Public Health 2018;15(2). https://doi.org/10.3390/ijerph15020206.

93. Field T, Diego M, Hernandez-Reif M. Massage therapy research. Dev Rev 2007; 27(1):75–89.

94. Gok Metin Z, Ozdemir L. The effects of aromatherapy massage and reflexology on pain and fatigue in patients with rheumatoid arthritis: a randomized controlled trial. Pain Manag Nurs 2016;17(2):140–9.

95. Field T, Diego M, Delgado J, et al. Rheumatoid arthritis in upper limbs benefits from moderate pressure massage therapy. Complement Ther Clin Pract 2013; 19(2):101–3.

96. Field T, Hernandez-Reif M, Seligman S, et al. Juvenile rheumatoid arthritis: benefits from massage therapy. J Pediatr Psychol 1997;22(5):607–17.

97. Otter S, Church A, Murray A, et al. The effects of reflexology in reducing the symptoms of fatigue in people with rheumatoid arthritis: a preliminary study. J Altern Complement Med 2010;16(12):1251–2.

98. Chunco LMT. The effects of massage on pain, stiffness, and fatigue levels associated with ankylosing spondylitis: a case study. Int J Ther Massage Bodywork 2011;4(1):12–7.

99. Romanowski MW, Špiritović M, Rutkowski R, et al. Comparison of deep tissue massage and therapeutic massage for lower back pain, disease activity, and functional capacity of ankylosing spondylitis patients: a randomized clinical pilot study. Evid Based Complement Altern Med 2017;2017. https://doi.org/10.1155/2017/9894128.

100. Roberts JA 4th, Mandl LA. Complementary and alternative medicine use in psoriatic arthritis patients: a review. Curr Rheumatol Rep 2020;22(11):81.

101. Abilash Kumar AK, Mohd QMQ, Ahmad ZAH, et al. Fracture-dislocation at C6-C7 level with quadriplegia after traditional massage in a patient with ankylosing spondylitis: a case report. Malays Orthop J 2017;11(2):75–7.

102. Zou G, Wang G, Li J, et al. Danger of injudicious use of tui-na therapy in ankylosing spondylitis. Eur Spine J 2017;26:1–3.

103. Ernst E. The safety of massage therapy. Rheumatology (Oxford) 2003;1101–6. https://doi.org/10.1093/rheumatology/keg306.

104. Egan M, Brosseau L, Farmer M, et al. Splints and orthosis for treating rheumatoid arthritis. Cochrane Database Syst Rev. 2001 Oct 23. https://doi.org/10.1002/14651858.CD004018.www.cochranelibrary.com.
105. Gijon-Nogueron G, Ramos-Petersen L, Ortega-Avila AB, et al. Effectiveness of foot orthoses in patients with rheumatoid arthritis related to disability and pain: a systematic review and meta-analysis. Qual Life Res 2018;27(12):3059–69.
106. Silva AC, Jones A, Silva PG, et al. Effectiveness of a night-time hand positioning splint in rheumatoid arthritis: a randomized controlled trial. J Rehabil Med 2008;40(9):749–54.
107. Grazio S, Grubišić F, Brnić V. Rehabilitation of patients with spondyloarthritis: a narrative review. Med Glas 2019;16(2):144–56.
108. Patience A, Helliwell PS, Siddle HJ. Focusing on the foot in psoriatic arthritis: pathology and management options. Expert Rev Clin Immunol 2018;14(1):21–8.
109. Shore A, Ansell BM. Juvenile psoriatic arthritis-an analysis of 60 cases. J Pediatr 1982;100(4):529–35.
110. Verhagen AP, Bierma-Zeinstra SMA, Boers M, et al. Balneotherapy for rheumatoid arthritis. Cochrane Database Syst Rev 2004;1. https://doi.org/10.1002/14651858.CD000518.
111. Cozzi F, Ciprian L, Carrara M, et al. Balneotherapy in chronic inflammatory rheumatic diseases—a narrative review. Int J Biometeorol 2018;62(12):2065–71.
112. Santos I, Cantista P, Vasconcelos C. Balneotherapy in rheumatoid arthritis—a systematic review. Int J Biometeorol 2016;60(8):1287–301.
113. Altan L, Bingöl Ü, Aslan M, et al. The effect of balneotherapy on patients with ankylosing spondylitis. Scand J Rheumatol 2006;35(4):283–9.
114. Urruela MA, Suarez-Almazor ME. Acupuncture in the treatment of rheumatic diseases. Curr Rheumatol Rep 2012;14(6):589–97.
115. Lee MS, Ernst E. Acupuncture for pain: an overview of Cochrane reviews. Chin J Integr Med 2011;17(3):187–9.
116. Kelly RB. Acupuncture for pain. Am Fam Physician 2009;80(5):89–96.
117. Seca S, Miranda D, Cardoso D, et al. Effectiveness of acupuncture on pain, physical function and health-related quality of life in patients with rheumatoid arthritis: a systematic review of quantitative evidence. Chin J Integr Med 2019;25(9):704–9.
118. Wang C, De Pablo P, Chen X, et al. Acupuncture for pain relief in patients with rheumatoid arthritis: a systematic review. Arthritis Care Res 2008;59(9):1249–56.
119. Lee MS, Shin BC, Ernst E. Acupuncture for rheumatoid arthritis: a systematic review. Rheumatology 2008;47(12):1747–53.
120. Seca S, Patrício M, Kirch S, et al. Effectiveness of acupuncture on pain, functional disability, and quality of life in rheumatoid arthritis of the hand: results of a double-blind randomized clinical trial. J Altern Complement Med 2019;25(1):86–97.
121. Lee JA, Son MJ, Choi J, et al. Bee venom acupuncture for rheumatoid arthritis: a systematic review of randomised clinical trials. BMJ Open 2014;4(11). https://doi.org/10.1136/bmjopen-2014-006140.
122. Attia AMM, Ibrahim FAA, Abd El-Latif NA, et al. Therapeutic antioxidant and anti-inflammatory effects of laser acupuncture on patients with rheumatoid arthritis. Lasers Surg Med 2016;48(5):490–7.
123. Adams ML, Arminio GJ. Non-pharmacologic pain management intervention. Clin Podiatr Med Surg 2008;25(3):409–29.

124. Marchetti G, Vittori A, Mascilini I, et al. Acupuncture for pain management in pediatric psoriatic arthritis: a case report. Acupunct Med 2020;23. https://doi.org/10.1177/0964528420920281.

125. Langhorst J, Klose P, Musial F, et al. Efficacy of acupuncture in fibromyalgia syndrome: a systematic review with a meta-analysis of controlled clinical trials. Rheumatology (Oxford) 2010;49(4):778–88.

126. Smith MT, Haythornthwaite JA. How do sleep disturbance and chronic pain inter-relate? Insights from the longitudinal and cognitive-behavioral clinical trials literature. Sleep Med Rev 2004;8(2):119–32.

127. Grabovac I, Haider S, Berner C, et al. Sleep quality in patients with rheumatoid arthritis and associations with pain, disability, disease duration, and activity. J Clin Med 2018;7(10):336.

128. Golenbiewski JT, Pisetsky DS. A holistic approach to pain management in the rheumatic diseases. Curr Treat Options Rheumatol 2019;5(1):1–10.

129. Goes ACJ, Reis LAB, Silva MBG, et al. Rheumatoid arthritis and sleep quality. Rev Bras Reumatol Engl Ed 2017;57(4):294–8.

130. Irwin MR, Olmstead R, Carrillo C, et al. Sleep loss exacerbates fatigue, depression, and pain in rheumatoid arthritis. Sleep 2012;35(4):537–43.

131. Wolfe F, Michaud K, Li T. Sleep disturbance in patients with rheumatoid arthritis: evaluation by medical outcomes study and visual analog sleep scales. J Rheumatol 2006;33(10):1942–51.

132. Tang NKY, Lereya ST, Boulton H, et al. Nonpharmacological treatments of insomnia for long-term painful conditions: a systematic review and meta-analysis of patient-reported outcomes in randomized controlled trials. Sleep 2015;38(11):1751–1764E.

133. Durcan L, Wilson F, Cunnane G. The effect of exercise on sleep and fatigue in rheumatoid arthritis: a randomized controlled study. J Rheumatol 2014;41(10):1966–73.

134. Latocha KM, Løppenthin KB, Østergaard M, et al. Cognitive behavioural therapy for insomnia in patients with rheumatoid arthritis: protocol for the randomised, single-blinded, parallel-group Sleep-RA trial. Trials 2020;21(1):440.

135. Troxel WM, Germain A, Buysse DJ. Clinical management of insomnia with brief behavioral treatment (BBTI). Behav Sleep Med 2012;10(4):266–79.

136. Leverment S, Clarke E, Wadeley A, et al. Prevalence and factors associated with disturbed sleep in patients with ankylosing spondylitis and non-radiographic axial spondyloarthritis: a systematic review. Rheumatol Int 2017;37(2):257–71.

137. Wong ITY, Chandran V, Li S, et al. Sleep disturbance in psoriatic disease: prevalence and associated factors. J Rheumatol 2017;44(9):1369–74.

138. Wadeley A, Clarke E, Leverment S, et al. Sleep in ankylosing spondylitis and non-radiographic axial spondyloarthritis: associations with disease activity, gender and mood. Clin Rheumatol 2018;37(4):1045–52.

139. Haugeberg G, Hoff M, Kavanaugh A, et al. Psoriatic arthritis: exploring the occurrence of sleep disturbances, fatigue, and depression and their correlates. Arthritis Res Ther 2020;22(1):1–10.

140. Gezer O, Batmaz İ, Sariyildiz MA, et al. Sleep quality in patients with psoriatic arthritis. Int J Rheum Dis 2017;20(9):1212–8.

141. Michelsen B, Fiane R, Diamantopoulos AP, et al. A comparison of disease burden in rheumatoid arthritis, psoriatic arthritis and axial spondyloarthritis. PLoS One 2015;10(4):1–11.

142. Sveaas SH, Dagfinrud H, Berg IJ, et al. High-intensity exercise improves fatigue, sleep, and mood in patients with axial spondyloarthritis: secondary analysis of a randomized controlled trial. Phys Ther 2020;100(8):1323–32.

143. Isik A, Koca SS, Ozturk A, et al. Anxiety and depression in patients with rheumatoid arthritis. Clin Rheumatol 2007;26(6):872–8.

144. Kotsis K, Voulgari PV, Tsifetaki N, et al. Anxiety and depressive symptoms and illness perceptions in psoriatic arthritis and associations with physical health-related quality of life. Arthritis Care Res 2012;64(10):1593–601.

145. Zhao S, Thong D, Miller N, et al. The prevalence of depression in axial spondyloarthritis and its association with disease activity: a systematic review and meta-analysis. Arthritis Res Ther 2018;20(1):1–9.

146. Rao JK, Mihaliak K, Kroenke K, et al. Use of complementary therapies for arthritis among patients of rheumatologists. Ann Intern Med 1999;131(6): 409–16.

147. Pittler MH, Brown EM, Ernst E. Static magnets for reducing pain: systematic review and meta-analysis of randomized trials. CMAJ 2007;177(7):736–42.

148. Segal NA, Toda Y, Huston J, et al. Two configurations of static magnetic fields for treating rheumatoid arthritis of the knee: a double-blind clinical trial. Arch Phys Med Rehabil 2001;82(10):1453–60.

149. Liao CC, Chen LR. Anterior and posterior fixation of a cervical fracture induced by chiropractic spinal manipulation in ankylosing spondylitis: a case report. J Trauma 2007;63(4):90–4.

150. Bonic EE, Stockwell CA, Kettner NW. Brain stem compression and atlantoaxial instability secondary to chronic rheumatoid arthritis in a 67-year-old female. J Manipulative Physiol Ther 2010;33(4):315–20.

Moving?

Make sure your subscription moves with you!

To notify us of your new address, find your **Clinics Account Number** (located on your mailing label above your name), and contact customer service at:

Email: journalscustomerservice-usa@elsevier.com

800-654-2452 (subscribers in the U.S. & Canada)
314-447-8871 (subscribers outside of the U.S. & Canada)

Fax number: 314-447-8029

Elsevier Health Sciences Division
Subscription Customer Service
3251 Riverport Lane
Maryland Heights, MO 63043

*To ensure uninterrupted delivery of your subscription, please notify us at least 4 weeks in advance of move.

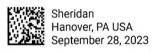